Nursing Homes from A-Z

Nursing Homes from A-Z

◆

A guide designed to educate residents and family members in navigating the complex environment of a nursing home

REYNOLDS C. CHAPMAN, B.S.

iUniverse, Inc.
New York Lincoln Shanghai

Nursing Homes from A-Z
A guide designed to educate residents and family members in navigating the complex environment of a nursing home

iUniverse books may be ordered through booksellers or by contacting:

iUniverse
2021 Pine Lake Road, Suite 100
Lincoln, NE 68512
www.iuniverse.com
1-800-Authors (1-800-288-4677)

Because of the dynamic nature of the Internet, any Web addresses or links contained in this book may have changed since publication and may no longer be valid.

ISBN: 978-0-595-45317-7 (pbk)
ISBN: 978-0-595-89631-8 (ebk)

Printed in the United States of America

International Standard Book Number:

Library of Congress Catalog Card Number: 2007903283

First Printing:

Contents

INTRODUCTION

How and when does an individual or a family member finally come to the realization that entering a long term care facility is the most appropriate placement for someone at this stage in their lives?

You have tried your best, for so long, to continue to function in your home despite numerous health concerns that have arisen in recent years. If you try to remain in an independent setting for too long, you run the risk of neglecting your physical well-being to the point of exhaustion, dehydration, significant weight loss, and possible skin breakdown. If your symptoms become severe enough, you may never fully recover.

On an emotional level, you may find that you are now going to feel lonelier than ever before as you realize that contact with family and friends will now be restricted. While neighbors, friends, and family members do their best to be supportive, some have difficulty observing a friend, neighbor, or family member deteriorate mentally and/or physically. They may want to suggest that you enter an assisted living facility or a long term care facility however, they do not risk hurting your feelings or making you angry.

On a cognitive level, while still living in your home, you may start misplacing items around the house, and in your frustration at not being able to locate certain items, you may find yourself blaming others for taking items from your home, only to find the item at a later time. It may be 10:00am and you may not be able to recall whether you had your breakfast or whether you have taken your prescribed medications to ensure your emotional and/or physical well-being. Many an elderly person has taken multiple doses of medications related to memory deficits that jeopardizes their health and may lead to injuries from falls.

Should you become weaker and possibly more confused, you will more than likely become a serious fall risk. There may come a time when you fall at home and cannot stand up without assistance. If you do not already subscribe to an in-home medical monitoring system, I would strongly suggest that you do as soon as possible. Without such a service, you may fall and find yourself spending long periods of time on the floor, and possibly seriously injured, for hours or days at a time.

On a financial level, as you become more cognitively impaired, you may find yourself neglecting your financial responsibilities. You may not remember to pay your monthly utilities bills and, as a result, run the risk of having your utilities turned off. When this happens, you may call a utility company and angrily complain that there must be some sort of mistake, when in fact you did not pay a utility bill. When your utilities are shut off, you can incur late fees that may put a strain on your finances. Should you find yourself in this situation, there are usually agencies that, for a fee, will manage your finances for you if you are having difficulty remembering to pay your monthly bills.

Have you noticed that others drivers are honking at you on a daily basis? You become convinced that they are the problem driver and not you. Remember, someone may contact the Department of Motor Vehicles and report you as a problem driver and you may be called by the Department of Motor Vehicles and be required to take another driver's test. Should you experience some or all of the above scenarios, you may be well entrenched in your crisis and find it quite difficult to resolve.

As a family member, when do you decide it is now time to place your loved one in a long term care facility? How long have you been telling yourself, "I'll do this for as long as I can"? How long have family members and friends been telling you that you are risking your physical and emotional well-being by trying to keep your loved one at home for so long? You continue to convince yourself that, as a caregiver, you can prevent your loved one's decline from happening if you make sure that your loved one is "never out of my sight". When your loved one starts wandering out of the house at all hours of the day related to their lack of safety awareness, secondary to some form of dementia, is a good time to start considering placement in a long term care facility and also if your spouse does not recognize you any longer.

At this point, you are now permitting your role as a caregiver to completely engulf every aspect of your life. Your loved one is now starting to leave the stove burners on and faucets running continuously and you are now following them around the house turning off the stove and faucets. What are you going to do with your loved one when you have to take a shower or bath and they must be out of your sight for a brief period of time?

Your loved one may now be experiencing sundowner's syndrome and is now sleeping more during the day and wandering aimlessly around the house at night if not trying to leaving your house. You are now following your loved one around the house at night to ensure their safety.

Before long, you are now exhausted most of your waking life. You are now more than likely neglecting your physical and emotional needs. You may find yourself becoming more temperamental toward your loved one, and as a result, find yourself becoming angry when they exhibit inappropriate behavior. You may become resentful that you had to change your entire lifestyle because you are now a full-time caregiver.

Deciding that it is the proper time for you to place your loved one in a long term care facility can be a very physical and emotional time in your life. Do not attempt to do it all on your own. Enlist the aid of family and friends, as well as, support groups and social service agencies in your community. The social worker in a long term care facility should be able to assist you in locating appropriate support groups and long term care facilities generally hold monthly Family Council Meetings that also can offer support during your adjustment period.

1

ASSESSMENT OF A NURSING HOME

When one must enter a nursing home for a short period of time or is going to become a permanent resident, it can be a confusing, frustrating ordeal. You will probably ask yourself "what do I do now" or "where do I start"? Be prepared to undergo a major change in your lifestyle. If you are fortunate enough to have family members close by, it would be of great benefit to enlist their emotional support and placement assistance.

Start your search by compiling a list of nursing homes in your local area and you may want to start with facilities that are close to family members to facilitate frequent visits. When you locate a nursing home, contact the Admissions office of the facility and schedule a tour of the facility. When scheduling a tour, try to have family members present because the more eyes you have observing the facility, the better. Schedule your tour at a time of day when the nursing home is likely to be the most active. A good time frame would be between 10:00am and 3:00pm so you can observe how active the residents are and how well groomed they are.

This is also a good opportunity to observe the staff to gain insight in to the various functions they perform as it relates to residents care needs and social interaction. Some of the things to look for while on your tour will include observing the residents who reside within the facility. Do they appear content, smiling, clean, and well groomed versus sleeping in lounge chairs and wheelchairs for extended period of time?

It would be of benefit to you and your family members if the tour included observing the lunch meal being served. You can observe how meals are served and if they appear nutritious. Are staff members assisting residents with their meals if they are having difficulty feeding themselves? Have some resident fallen asleep at the dining table, and if so, is the staff attempting to intervene to ensure that a resident is aroused, encouraged, and assisted with completing their meals?

Look around to assess the cleanliness of the facility. Look in the corners. Look in the dining room to see if there is food and/or liquids present on the floor that may have been ignored by staff. Do the carpets appear clean, vacuumed, and stain-free? Does the vinyl appear clean and free from spills?

Observe for disorganization in the environment such as linen and food carts interfering with the normal flow of resident and visitor traffic. Observe the nurses station. Does it appear organized? Are there charts scattered about and is paperwork stacked on top of each other? If so, this is one way a resident's paperwork may get filed in the wrong chart. Looking at these issues will give you some insight into how organized or disorganized the staff may be as it relates to the delivery of services and an organized nurses' station will minimize paperwork errors. While on your tour, do you smell the odor of urine and/or feces? While this occurs from time to time related to incontinent residents, most nursing homes do their best to keep odors to a minimum so as not to dissuade a resident from being admitted to their nursing home, especially if the census is low. While on your tour, should you smell the odor of urine and/or feces, politely inquire of your tour guide as to the source of the odor.

Request to view a private room versus a semi-private room to assess how much space each resident is afforded and whether the room will accommodate your furnishings. Observe carefully when doing this because some rooms are designed in such a manner where one resident may be afforded more space than their roommate in a semi-private room. In a semi-private room, another important factor is where the bathroom door is located. Is it at the foot of your bed or that of your roommate? This is a good time to inquire as to what possessions/furnishings you will be permitted to have in your room. Inquire as to whether a situation could possibly arise that would require a resident to vacate a private room and have to relocate to a semi-private room. I have encountered angry and frustrated residents and family members who were not very pleased with having to vacate a private room.

While on a tour of a nursing home, request to meet a representative from the activity department and inquire as to the various activities the facility has to offer so that you can be assured the activities offered will meet your social needs, as well as, being mentally stimulating. Also meet with the Clinical Dietician to assess whether the facility is able to meet your dietary needs and possible dietary restrictions related to solid foods, liquids, and feeding tubes, also known as "peg tubes".

Be sure to inquire as to where or on what unit within the nursing home you would be placed should you be admitted to their facility. While some nursing homes adequately screen potential admissions to ensure that a resident is placed in the most appropriate area of the facility as it relates to their medical needs, direct care needs, cognitive status, and behavioral deficits, some nursing homes do not. At times, residents may be placed in an area of the nursing home that meets the needs of the facility and not necessarily the needs of the resident.

A great number of nursing homes have units specifically designated for residents diagnosed with dementia. Many geriatric individuals and their family members have a great deal of difficulty accepting/coping with a diagnosis of dementia. As a resident diagnosed with dementia or a health care surrogate of a resident diagnosed with dementia, the resident will more than likely be placed on the dementia unit. If this is the case, please do not initially become angry because this is not necessarily a bad thing. Dementia units offer activities that are structured to meet the activity and social needs of cognitively impaired residents.

If a cognitively impaired resident is placed on a unit with cognitively intact residents, they will feel out of place and will have difficulty interacting appropriately with their peers. If placement on a dementia unit is indicated while on a tour of a nursing home, request to see and observe the dementia unit and then draw your own conclusions.

There are various stages of dementia and as a protective family member or health care surrogate, you want to do your best to assure that your loved one or resident is not placed on a dementia unit prematurely. If a resident diagnosed with mild dementia is placed on a unit with residents that are diagnosed with moderate or severe dementia, they may cognitively decompensate at a faster rate than if placed with more appropriate residents.

If you have any concerns about where you will be placed within a nursing home when admitted now is the time to speak up. Once a resident is already placed on a unit in a nursing home, it is my feeling that the facility may have the "upper hand" as to if, when, and where a resident may be relocated to another unit of the nursing home.

While on your tour, inquire as to whether the nursing home has a "bed hold" policy should a resident require hospitalization and it is their desire to return to the same room and bed when discharged from the hospital. Be sure to ask the Admissions Coordinator what your financial responsibility to the nursing home will be, if any, should you request the nursing home hold your same room and bed for you while you are in a hospital. Failure to inquire about a nursing home's bed hold policy may result in you and/or family members scrambling to locate another nursing home when a resident is discharge ready from the hospital. As a resident in a nursing home and you must relocate to another nursing home for whatever reason, meet with your assigned social worker for assistance with this matter.

While on your tour of a nursing home, request to see the nursing homes annual survey results to assess the number and severity of deficiencies they received during their annual inspection and their plan of correction.

2

ACTIVITIES

As an individual about to be admitted to a nursing home you may be somewhat overwhelmed as to how you are going to spend your time while awake within the nursing home. Once in a nursing home, you will not be able to pursue some activities of interest you enjoyed prior to placement in the nursing home. You may obsess about how you are going to obtain the sensory/social stimulation that you need, enjoy, and benefit from.

All nursing homes are mandated by governing agencies to provide a variety of activities that are structured to meet a resident's current medical, cognitive, and physical limitations. Once you are in a nursing home, be sure to obtain a monthly calendar of all the activities offered and select activities of interest. Plan on meeting with a representative from the activity department to share your specific activity interests and become educated as to how the activity department is going to interact with you as it relates to meeting your social needs.

As a resident or family member of a resident, ensure the activity department is doing their best to encourage and assist residents with attending structured activities. When visiting, some family members often find their loved ones sleeping in bed, a chair, or their wheelchairs when they arrive. When this occurs, family members often feel that the activity department is not doing their best to ensure that their loved one is being encouraged to attend and assisted to structured activities. If this is the case, as a family member, vary your visiting hours during the week to assess whether this pattern occurs at any particular time of the day. If this becomes a chronic issue, request to meet with the Director of Activities and the nursing staff to hopefully resolve this issue. If necessary, be sure to consult with the nursing staff to ensure that a resident is afforded rest periods and/or naps during the day so a resident may have the energy to attend and participate in activities of interest.

While a nursing home may offer a wide variety of structured and individual activities, family members often have difficulty accepting that their loved one is refusing to attend activities. They often say "make them go" or "don't ask them if they want to go, just take them". This approach may seem the easiest for family members however they must remember that residents have rights as it relates to not being coerced to attend activities offered by the nursing home. At times, I have observed activity department staff wheeling a resident to an activity, and the whole time, the resident was loudly protesting and insisting they did not want to attend the activity.

Structured activities should be held in a room or area of the nursing home that provides adequate lighting, ventilation, space, equipment and supplies. When activities involving foods are held, the activity department staff should take into account the food preferences and dietary restrictions of the activity participants and provide assistance and adaptive equipment as needed.

Some residents in nursing homes prefer individual activities as opposed to group activities. As a resident in a nursing home and you prefer individual activities, meet with the activity director or leader and share your desire for individual activities and what activities you prefer. Identify what supplies and equipment you will need and request that the activity department provide the supplies you will require to enjoy an activity of your choice.

A resident's individualized comprehensive Activity Care Plan should be based upon goals, interests, and preferences of the resident. The care plan should also identify how the nursing home will provide activities to help residents attain any set goals and who is responsible for implementation.

3

ADVANCED MEDICAL DIRECTIVES

Advanced Medical Directives are legal documents that one completes to educate family, friends, and health care providers of your wishes as it relates to the delivery of health care services. The following documents are examples of the most common advanced medical directives.

LIVING WILL: is an advanced medical directive that educates health care providers as to what medical intervention they are to initiate as it relates to terminal illness and life sustaining medical procedures. One can obtain Living Will forms from a nursing home, their attorney, the Internet or agencies that provide legal documents however, you may prefer to author your own living will that is more specific in nature. An important aspect of a Living Will that one must keep in mind is that an individual must have cognitive capacity to sign a living will. The issue of cognitive capacity is generally addressed by an individual's personal physician, their assigned physician in a nursing home or the court system (see chapter related to Capacity).

When interpreting a living will, be sure you pay close attention to the wording in the document. Most of the generic versions of living wills that I have had to read and interpret indicate that the resident must have a terminal condition or is in a vegetative state and a physician has indicated that it is their medical opinion that the resident is not expected to emerge from the vegetative state for the living will to be activated.

DO NOT RESUSCITATE: is commonly referred to as a **DNR**. This advanced medical directive instructs health care providers to withhold Cardio-Pulmonary Resuscitation **(CPR)** in the event you experience cardiac and/or respiratory arrest. Once again, an individual must have cognitive capacity to sign a DNR form and said form must be signed by a physician.

If it is your preference to be DNR status, it would help to carry a copy of your DNR form with you when you leave your home or a nursing home in the event you experience cardiac and/or respiratory arrest when you are not in a medical facility such as when you go shopping or out to eat at restaurants. It is usually the responsibility of the social worker in a long term care facility to meet with a resident who has capacity to make their own health care decisions or an appointed health care surrogate to provide education related to advanced medical directives and their right to determine their **CODE STATUS**. DNR means CPR will be withheld and FULL CODE means CPR will be initiated in the event a resident in a long term care facility experiences cardiac and/ or respiratory arrest.

Most of the nursing staff that I have worked with in long term care facilities shutter at the idea of a resident being FULL CODE status. A fear that staff may have is the possibility of causing injuries to an elderly resident while performing CPR and this can occur. ALL health care employees must never lose sight of the fact that regardless of their concerns or fears, an individual's choice of code status is their right, regardless of how they feel about performing CPR on a geriatric resident.

I have heard comments by nursing staff that if a FULL CODE resident experiences cardiac and/or respiratory arrest on their shift, they will execute what is called a "slow-code", meaning that there will not be any rush to initiate CPR. I have also heard that if a staff member is in the room of a FULL CODE resident and they are the only witness to the resident's cardiac and/or respiratory arrest, they should leave the room, close the door, and not say anything.

Another misperception of some nursing staff in long term care facilities, to include management, is to perceive a DNR order to also mean **D0 NOT HOSPITALIZE**. These are two very different advanced medical directives. When I have witnessed a resident physically deteriorating and felt they may benefit from hospitalization, I have mentioned it to a Nurse Manager, an ADON, and a DON, only to be told that the resident is DNR status. Residents in nursing homes may very well be DNR status, however, they would also benefit from brief hospitalization related to fractures, head trauma, seizures, etc.

DO NOT RESUSCITATE only applies to whether CPR is to be initiated or withheld in the event a resident experiences cardiac and/or respiratory arrest. Whether you are an individual about to be admitted to a long term care facility or you are a family member that must now place a loved one in a long care facility, be sure that you have a conversation with nursing management as it relates to their perception of DNR versus DO NOT HOSPITALIZE.

HEALTH CARE SURROGATE DESIGNATION: is an advanced medical directive that appoints an individual or a group of individuals such as multiple family members to act on your behalf as it relates to the delivery of medical care only in the event you have been declared by a physician or the court system as lacking capacity to make your own health care decisions. Most health care surrogate designation forms generally suggest you to appoint a primary health care surrogate, as well as, an alternate health care surrogate in the event the primary health care surrogate cannot be contacted, or they do not wish to serve in this capacity any longer.

We must remember that lacking capacity to make one's own medical decisions can be a temporary situation related to certain medical complications such as post-operative anesthesia, unconsciousness, coma, or head trauma. It is very important, especially for the geriatric population, to appoint a health care surrogate when major surgery is planned in the event one experiences a medical emergency during surgery that results in further physical and/or cognitive decline. We must also remember that once an individual regains cognitive capacity, as determined by a physician or the court system, they are now entitled to exercise their right to make their own health care decisions.

Appointing a health care surrogate that you trust and are convinced will honor your wishes as it relates to delivery of health care is one of the most important decisions that you will ever have to make. Some individuals appoint several health care surrogates with equal authorization, such as adult children, that can eventually cause numerous conflicts between a resident in a long term care facility, their family, and the staff of a long term care facility. If your multiple health care surrogates are unable to come to a collective agreement as it relates to making health care decisions for you, it could lead to your medical decline by being denied appropriate medical interventions. That is why it is important to do your best to appoint one primary health care surrogate, as well as, an alternate health care surrogate.

We must remember that an individual appointed their primary and alternate health care surrogates while they still had capacity to make his/her own health care decisions. As long as an individual has capacity to make their own health care decisions, they have the right to change their appointed primary and alternate health care surrogates as often as they feel the need too. Once an individual is declared as lacking capacity to make their own health care decisions, they can no longer change or appoint new health care surrogates.

Being appointed a primary health care surrogate for someone is a voluntary role. If for whatever reason you find that you are no longer able to fulfill the role as primary health care surrogate, you may transfer your authority to the alternate health care surrogate appointed by an individual while they had capacity to make their own health care decisions. If an individual lacks capacity to make their own health care decisions, their appointed primary and alternate health care surrogates cannot transfer their health care decision making authority to someone that was not appointed as a health care surrogate by an individual when they had cognitive capacity to make their own health care decisions. For an alternate health care surrogate to be able to relinquish their role as a health care surrogate to someone not appointed by an individual while they still had capacity to make their own health care decisions, a form called Health Care Proxy Designation must be completed.

<u>HEALTH CARE PROXY DESIGNATION</u>: When an individual lacks capacity to make their own health care decisions and they have not appointed a health care surrogate, an individual must be appointed to make health care decisions for the individual. A health care proxy designation is very specific as to who has the first opportunity to be appointed a resident's Health Care Proxy.

Generally a surviving spouse would be the first consideration as a health care proxy. If a spouse cannot serve in this capacity, the next appointees are generally adult children of the incapacitated resident. The resident's social worker generally contacts the adult children to assess who will be the primary health care proxy. Once an agreement amongst the adult children has been reached as to who will be appointed a resident's health care proxy, the social worker should require a letter signed by the remaining adult children indicating they have no objection to a particular adult sibling being appointed the primary health care proxy. The social worker should also have the appointed Health Care Proxy sign a form related to acceptance of this role. The letter should then be placed in a resident's medical record.

This approach minimizes confusion as to who actually is the appointed health care proxy for a resident. If a resident has no surviving relatives, a good friend who knows the individual well may be appointed as a health care proxy. If there is absolutely no one who can be appointed as health care proxy for a cognitively impaired resident, guardianship proceedings are generally the last resort. The social worker in the nursing home is generally the one to initiate guardianship proceedings on behalf of the resident and the nursing home. Guardianship can be a very lengthy, grueling process, therefore, if it can be avoided, the better off for all involved.

<u>DURABLE POWER OF ATTORNEY</u>: This advanced medical directive generally appoints someone who will be authorized to manage your finances should you lack cognitive and/or physical capacity to manage your own finances. If a resident did not appoint a power of attorney while they had capacity to manage their own financial affairs, you, as a family member, will more than likely have to initiate guardianship proceedings.

Should this occur, you should retain the services of an attorney who specializes in Elder Law. It may cost you money but, in the long run, it will save you quite a bit of time and aggravation. If you find yourself being appointed a legal guardian for another individual, be sure you fully understand the legal ramifications and expectations of you while fulfilling your role as a legal guardian.

Prior to appointing a health care surrogate or durable power of attorney, plan to meet with potential candidates and discuss your wishes as it relates to future medical care and/or financial assistance. Over the years, I have observed numerous health care surrogates, health care proxies, and legal guardians make medical and financial decisions for their resident that were not in compliance with the residents signed advanced medical directives. Often, health care decision makers experience guilt if they do not approve a medical procedure for a resident, regardless of the wording in their resident's advanced medical directives.

As an appointed health care surrogate, health care proxy, or a legal guardian, should you find yourself making medical decisions for another individual that are based on what you want for the resident, and not necessarily what the resident instructed in their advanced medical directives, it is time for you to seriously consider relinquishing your role as a health care decision maker for a resident in a nursing home.

4

BILLING ISSUES

Ensuring that your monthly bill for services rendered by a nursing home is accurate can often be a frustrating, tedious process for most residents, family members and Power of Attorneys, therefore, ALWAYS review your monthly billing statement. Sometimes, residents in long term care facilities, whether it be a nursing home or an assisted living facility, are billed for items and services they did not receive such as medications, incontinence supplies, oxygen or dietary supplements such as Ensure or Boost to name a few. I think it is a gross misuse of a resident's finances when oxygen tanks remain in a resident's room long after an order was received to discontinue the use of oxygen and they are still being billed for it.

If you have a telephone in your room in a nursing home, examine the monthly bill closely or have a family assist you with this task because there are instances when staff members would not hesitate to make long distance telephone calls from your telephone. Be sure that any charges for long distance calls are for calls that you have initiated. If you find questionable charges on your monthly telephone statement, meet with the nurse manager assigned to you or your loved one and be sure to have the monthly telephone statement with you. Together, the both of you should be able to determine where the call was placed, the day of the week the call was placed, as well as, the time of day the call was made. With this information, the nurse manager should be able to cross reference staffing schedules to identify on what shift the call was placed and what staff members were assigned to work at the time an unauthorized long distance call was placed.

If as a resident in a nursing home, you generally do not make long distance telephone calls, request that the facility or the telephone company place a long distance block on your telephone. This rarely happens but it does from time to time.

If a resident in a nursing home is incontinent of bowel and/or bladder, a resident generally has the right to furnish their own incontinence supplies or they can request that the nursing home furnish incontinence supplies that will be included on your monthly billing statement. If you prefer to have the facility furnish your incontinence supplies, during the admissions process, be sure to inquire as to the cost of the incontinence supplies they will be furnishing. If as a resident in a nursing home, you receive regular visits from friends and/or family members, it would be worth your while to furnish your own incontinence supplies because most nursing home will more then likely will mark up the price of supplies they furnish. Another benefit to furnishing your own incontinence supplies allows you to keep better controls over how many briefs are actually being used in a specific period of time. If you furnish your own incontinence supplies, be sure you do not run out of them because if this occurs, you will be issued briefs by the nursing home until you replenish your supply and will be billed for them.

If you are cognitively intact and the nursing home furnishes your incontinence briefs, you should be able to assess approximately how many incontinence briefs you generally require during the monthly billing period. If you are a family member of a resident in a nursing home and you provide the resident's incontinence supplies, you can, and very well should, meet with the staff to determine how many briefs you should deliver to the nursing home on a monthly basis. If you begin to notice that you are running out of incontinence supplies prematurely, meet with your assigned nurse and inquire as to why this is occurring. I mention this because there may be some caregivers that do not want to walk any farther that they have too to obtain an incontinence brief for a resident, therefore, they may use your incontinence supplies for your roommate and/or other residents in the nursing home.

Be sure that when you must meet with someone in a nursing home related to questionable billing charges on your monthly statement make certain that you meet with the most appropriate individual in the nursing home. It will not be productive to discuss billing issues with the nursing or dietary staff. Discuss questionable billing charges with your nurse manager, the Director of Nursing, the Administrator, and the manager of the billing department.

On a final note, as it relates to billing issues, be sure that your monthly billing statement is **ITEMIZED** and you are not just given a total amount of monthly charges. Without an itemized monthly billing statement, it deprives you of your right to examine the bill for accuracy and to be reassured that you are not paying for goods and services you did not receive.

5

CAPACITY TO MAKE HEALTH CARE DECISIONS

When you hear the terms "**Capacity**" and "**Lacks Capacity**", this generally refers to an individual's ability or inability to make reasonable and realistic health care decisions for themselves when the need arises that are generally related to dementia, medical issues, and/or mental health issues. This is such an important issue because being able to make one's own health care decisions is rooted in resident's rights and will be discussed in a later chapter.

It is so important for the admitting physician or ARNP to address a resident's cognitive capacity to make their own health care decisions as this information gives staff guidance as to who is making health care decisions for a resident and also to ensure that resident's rights are protected.

The issue of capacity is very important as to how it impacts a resident in a nursing home. As nursing home staff and family members, we must keep in mind that informing a resident that their right to make their own health care decisions is being forfeited secondary to their medical, cognitive, or mental health status can induce frustration, denial, and anger for a resident to the point they may refuse care. This will be expanded upon in the chapter related to mental health issues.

When meeting with the physician or ARNP, be sure as to inquire as to the criteria they follow when addressing capacity. If your loved one in a nursing home is deemed to lack capacity to make their own health care decisions, be sure you request this medical determination in writing as you may need to share this information with other health care providers and also to assess whether an appointed health care surrogate's role is now activated.

We must remember that lacking capacity to make our own health care decisions may be a temporary condition due to a wide variety of medical conditions. It is imperative that nursing homes employ educated, experienced, observant, and motivated staff as it relates to residents care needs. They must get to know their residents' very well as it relates to residents medical and cognitive status, as well as dietary and mood/behavioral deficits.

Should staff members in a nursing home suspect that a resident who lacks capacity to make their own health care decisions now appears to be making more reasonable, realistic, health care decisions for themselves, the staff have an ethical and professional responsibility to discuss this with a resident's physician or assigned ARNP to assess whether a resident's right to make their own health care decisions can be restored.

Given the impact that lacking capacity may have on certain residents in nursing homes as a health care surrogate, health care proxy, durable power of attorney, or a legal guardian, do your best to meet with the resident to tactfully discuss their health care needs and do your best to enlist their support in permitting you to assist them with making reasonable health care decisions.

I am well aware that the terms "realistic" and "reasonable" are open to a wide variety of interpretations, therefore, if your interpretation of these terms differ from that of the medical staff in the nursing home, be sure, you make time to meet with the physician and/or the ARNP to share your thoughts and interpretations.

6

CARE PLAN CONFERENCE

All nursing homes are mandated by governing agencies to schedule and conduct care plan conferences for all residents in their facility shortly after admission and at least on a quarterly basis thereafter. Typically, the initial care plan conference is generally scheduled no later than the twenty first day after admission to a nursing home. Staff members generally assigned to a care plan team includes the Care Plan Coordinator, the Nurse Manager, Social Worker, Dietician, and Activity Leader. It would be wise for a Care Plan Team to invite direct care staff to the care plan conference because they spend almost all of their working hours providing direct care to residents and they can be a wealth of knowledge as it relates to a resident's care needs, mood, and behavior. Sometimes this does not occur because the care plan coordinator may feel that there may not be sufficient time to conduct all the care plan conferences scheduled for that day.

Once a care plan conference is scheduled, a resident should receive a written invitation to attend their care plan conference that states the date, time, and where the care plan conference will be held. A resident's appointed health care surrogate, which is usually a family member, should also receive an invitation as well, however, it is the residents right to invite whomever they choose to attend their care plan conference. Sometimes residents do not want their health care information shared with family members for their own reasons. In some nursing homes, a resident who lacks capacity to make their own health care decisions are not extended an invitation to their care plan conference because, due to their cognitive status, the care plan team may feel they would not understand the information that is being discussed and/or a resident may exhibit anxious/agitated behavior related to the information being discussed.

Whether you are a resident, a family member, or health care surrogate, the care plan conference is your best opportunity to be able to meet with all the medical disciplines involved in your care or the care of your loved one. As soon as you receive an invitation to attend a care plan conference, be sure that you confirm with the social worker whether you are able or unable to attend the care plan conference. If you plan on attending, get a pen and pad and start writing down all the questions and concerns you may have as it relates to the care a resident receives. Remember, this is your time to gain knowledge and insight into your health care needs, prognosis, and Plan of Care or that of a family member.

All members of a Care Plan Team are required to author a Care Plan that should be individualized for every resident depending on their health care needs, cognitive status, activity pursuits, dietary needs, mood/behavioral deficits, as well as, short or long term placement plans for a resident. Each individualized care plan outlines what deficit is identified, a time frame to eliminate or minimize a deficit, and what approaches staff will initiate to hopefully eliminate or minimize an identifiable deficit a resident may be experiencing and/or exhibiting.

This is your time to review your individualized care plans and hopefully have them explained to you in a manner you are able to comprehend. Should you ever feel that a member of a care plan team is rushing you during the meeting, politely remind them that this is your only opportunity to be able to meet with all the members of your care plan team at one sitting. I have attended care plan conferences that were scheduled fifteen minutes apart. While this time frame may be appropriate for residents that lack capacity and their health care surrogate or family members are not planning to attend, however, when a cognitively intact resident or a health care surrogate plans on attending a care plan conference, the fifteen minute time frame is radically insufficient. There is just so much information to cover in such a short period of time. Should you require more time to learn about your medical condition, prognosis, and plan of care than the fifteen minutes that may be allotted, contact the care plan coordinator and request more time be allotted to your care plan conference. If they resist or refuse to allot more time for you at your care plan conference, schedule a meeting with the Director of Nursing and insist that you be given more time at your care plan conference to learn more about your medical needs and plan of care.

After the initial care plan conference is scheduled, future care plan conferences are scheduled on a quarterly basis. An exception to this rule is if you are in a nursing home on a Medicare unit (to be discussed in a later chapter), your care plan conferences will be more frequent. Another exception to this rule is what is referred to as a "significant change" care plan conference. These conferences are scheduled when a resident in a nursing home makes a significant improvement in their health care status or a significant decline in their health care status.

While attending a care plan conference, you will more than likely hear the term "**MDS**". It means "Minimum Data Set " which is a document that is completed by all disciplines of the care plan team that assist in authoring individualized care plans for a resident. The MDS is also a wealth of information as it relates to a resident's advanced medical directives, cognitive status, mood and/or behavioral deficits, dietary needs, skin condition, frequency of incontinence, the extent of direct care required and so much more.

When attending a care plan conference, have someone explain every aspect of the MDS to you in a manner you comprehend. Do not let members of a care plan team confuse and/or overwhelm you with complex medical terms and if there is something you do not fully comprehend ask for an explanation that you can comprehend. Do not permit the care plan team to rush you during the care plan conference. If they do, stand your ground and insist that you are not leaving the care plan conference until all your concerns are addressed. Do not leave the meeting with unanswered questions/concerns. Remember, the Care Plan Conference is **YOUR** time. The Care Plan Team may just have to learn how to better schedule their time so as afford a resident or health care surrogate adequate time at a Care Plan Conference.

7

CONFLICT RESOLUTION

While I acknowledge there are publications entirely devoted to conflict resolution, it is my intention to share some basic elements of conflict resolution as it relates to nursing homes that should enable a resident and/or family member to implement basic approaches as conflicts arise. Conflicts with the care one receive will arise from time to time and how the conflict is handled will certainly affect the outcome of the conflict.

As a resident or family member of a resident in a nursing home, should you present as angry, hostile, demanding, or insulting during a conflict with nursing home staff it will certainly jeopardize the outcome of a conflict. Another approach/attitude to avoid is the mindset of "it's my way or no way". A resident must remember that when they were admitted to a nursing home, at that point, they entrusted their care to the staff of the nursing home. Education and experience has taught me to believe that rather than trying to "win" a conflict, all parties involved should strive to reach a compromise related to alleviating the conflict that all parties will be comfortable with.

I have observed residents and family members' subject staff members to verbal abuse, anger, and excessive demanding behavior. If as a resident or family member, you believe taking this approach will get you want you want, think again. When staff members are subjected to this sort of treatment, they often become emotionally hurt and defensive, and generally consider the source of the abuse as unrealistic/unreasonable and often feel that there is nothing they can do to satisfy the abuser. Should you as a resident or family member become abusive to staff members, do not be surprised if you do not see the staff member as often as you used too because they are now doing their best to avoid you and will generally only interact with you when they have too. Being verbally abusive toward staff will only threaten any positive relationship the staff is attempting to establish with a resident or family member of a resident in a nursing home.

I am fully aware of how hard it may be for some folks to "bite their tongue" when they are not pleased, especially if they feel they are receiving poor medical care. If as a resident and/or family member of a resident in a nursing home, you find yourself having to address a conflict with staff, please take time to be as calm as possible and logically assess how you are going to initiate and conduct yourself during the conflict resolution process. By adopting this approach, I cannot help but feel that most of the time, you will observe a more positive and timely response from staff to the concerns you have addressed.

After repeated attempts to resolve a conflict with nursing staff without success, request a conference with the Director Nursing and the Administrator of the nursing home. An Administrator may be receptive to the concept of compromise because they may have more difficulty meeting the budget if a resident relocates to another nursing home because conflict resolution was not successful.

If after meeting with the director of Nursing and the Administrator, you are still not satisfied with the outcome of a conflict, contact your Ombudsman's office and file a formal complaint (see chapter related to the Ombudsman).

8

DIETARY NEEDS AND MEALS

When searching for a nursing home, be sure to meet with the certified dietary manager and the Registered Dietician to ensure that the nursing home will be able to meet your dietary and feeding needs. There is such a wide variety of prescribed diets in nursing homes, therefore, meeting the dietary needs of a resident should not be a problem. Prescribed diets in nursing homes generally include a regular diet, chopped diet, cardiac diet, diabetic diet, renal diets, pureed diet, liquids only diet, thickened liquids, and feeding tubes, also known as peg tubes.

From a medical perspective, it is very important to assess a resident's risk of aspiration when drinking thin liquids. Assessment of a resident's risk of aspiration should include consultations between the physician and ARNP, the Clinical Dietician, and the speech therapist. If it is determined that a resident in a nursing home is at risk for aspiration on thin liquids, they will more than likely be prescribed "thickened liquids" which is usually a powder that is added to thin liquids to thicken the liquid to a desired texture or consistency to reduce the risk of aspiration. If you have to drink thickened liquids, do not let them sit around very long as they have a tendency to thicken even more when they sit for extended periods of time. Thickened liquids can be quite difficult for some residents to swallow when they are mixed properly and when the liquids continue to thicken some residents cannot drink them at all. As a resident in a nursing home and you have capacity to make your own health care decisions, you should be able to reject certain dietary restrictions as long as you comprehend and accept the possible medical risks involved. Should this be the case, meet with the Registered Dietician and discuss this further.

Nursing homes generally provide menus for residents to select their food preferences. Residents with certain dietary restrictions will usually receive menus that are "customized" for their particular dietary restriction. Menus can usually be completed on a monthly, weekly, or daily basis. Some residents in nursing homes prefer to complete weekly menus as this affords a resident the opportunity to change their food preferences more often. It is very important that all staff in nursing homes become familiar with residents who have dietary restrictions so that a resident does not receive food/liquid items that may compromise their medical status. Do not assume that the dietary department that prepare meal trays are going to always prepare meal trays properly. Liquids may not be thickened as they should or a resident may receive food items they did not order or may have an allergy too.

During the assessment of a resident's dietary needs, it is so important to inquire as to whether the resident has food allergies that all staff should be made aware of. All nursing homes should have some form of quality control measures in place to ensure that the correct food/liquids items are placed on the food trays prior to it being placed in food carts to be delivered to residents within the facility. Residents in a nursing home generally have the option of having their meals in a central dining room as opposed to eating their meals in the dining room on their assigned unit or in their room.

The dietary department in a nursing home is one of the most difficult to operate. Residents and family members generally lack insight/knowledge into the number of regular meals and special diets that a dietary department must produce on a daily basis. Another hardship for some dietary departments in nursing homes are meals that must be prepared earlier or later than normally scheduled meal times related to medical issues or a resident may have a scheduled appointment out of the facility and will require their meal to be delivered before the appointment or when they return to the nursing home.

Given the number of meals that are prepared in a nursing home kitchen on a daily basis, please do not become too impatient or angry if occasionally a meal is late in arriving. However, if this becomes a chronic problem, be sure to meet with the dietary department manager to hopefully resolve this issue.

A complaint generally heard in nursing homes is the food usually arrives cold and this has a tendency to upset some folks. This may occur more often to residents who eat their meals in their room or a communal dining room on a particular unit within the nursing home because food arrives in meal carts that may sit in a hallway for an extended period of time. Most nursing homes utilize special type of plates that are designed to retain heat so that meals remain hotter for a longer period of time. Another option is to have your meals in the main dining room of the nursing home where the food is generally served off a serving line and may be hotter. As a resident in a nursing home, should you receive a hot meal that is now cold, request that the staff heat the meal in a microwave oven or politely request that the cold meal be returned to the kitchen and order a hot meal.

During the admissions process, be sure to confirm whether a resident will be charged for meals that they did not receive such as when they are in a hospital or leaving the nursing home with family members for specific or extended periods of time.

If you must leave a nursing home for extended periods of time and you do not have to pay for meals you have missed, be sure that you examine your monthly billing statement to ensure that you were not charged for the missed meals. This is very important because some staff members in nursing homes may not be aware that a resident is out of the facility and may continue to add charges to your monthly statement. Many nursing homes offer meal plans that are set at a certain price regardless of how often you eat their meals so be sure to inquire as to a nursing homes policy related to meals.

Some residents in a nursing home may require their meal tray to be properly set-up for them whether it is related to medical, cognitive, or visual deficits. Whether you prefer to have your meals served in your room, in the dining room on your unit, or in the main dining room, at times it can be very difficult to manage your meal tray independently. For a resident who has paralysis of an upper extremity related to a stroke, it can be very difficult to open cartons of milk or juice, peel a banana, open and butter a slice of bread, and open a container of jelly to name a few.

When this occurs, it can be a very frustrating, humiliating, and demoralizing experience for a resident. It may be a catalyst for a resident to start focusing to much on their cognitive and/or medical deficits which often exacerbate symptoms of depression such as feelings of helplessness/hopelessness, as well as possible weight loss. When a blind or severely visually impaired resident is served their meal the staff should educate the resident as to where the food items on their plate are located using the face of a clock as an analogy.

As a staff member in a nursing home, whether or not you are responsible for the delivery of meal trays, it is your duty to assist a resident having difficulty managing their meal tray or reporting this information to the appropriate staff so they may be more observant of residents having difficulty managing their meal trays.

Some residents that are cognitively impaired require constant encouragement and cueing to complete their meals. They often become distracted during their meal, may forget they are eating, and subsequently abandoning their meal. Staff are to remain in the dining room to observe residents during meal times to encourage and cue residents to complete their meals but also to observe for any medical emergencies that may arise such as a resident choking on food or aspirating liquids, or residents who may be exhibiting behavioral deficits that may interfere with other residents who are trying to enjoy their meals.

As a family member or a health care surrogate for a resident in a nursing home and they require assistance with their meals, I would encourage you to visit during meal times and observe whether the staff is providing the assistance residents may require to complete their meals and do not with their meals and may return a resident's meal tray to the food cart prematurely.

Nursing homes are mandated to serve nutritious meals and to ensure that residents receive the proper amount of calories. Should you become concerned as to whether a resident is receiving the proper amount of calories, meet with the nurse manager and request that a resident be weighed weekly for a period of time and monitor/record any changes in a resident's weight. Residents often find the amount of food being served at meal times is overwhelming. Providing a resident does not have a medical condition that would be contraindicated, they can request "small portion" meals. Just as some resident lose weight when in a nursing home, others gain weight. As a resident, be careful here because if you gain to much weight, it may now require the assistance of two direct care aides, as opposed to, one. If a resident gains a considerable amount of weight, they may not be able to independently transfer from a chair to a standing position or be able to get themselves in and out of bed. If you hear nursing staff mention the use of a **"Hoyer Lift"** to get you in and out of bed, watch out. This piece of equipment may be somewhat intimidating for some residents in nursing homes. A resident can minimize their need of a Hoyer Lift by managing their weight.

Residents often tire of food served in a nursing home because they are not accustomed to what they may consider institutional cooking and may miss foods they previously enjoyed. As a friend or family member, take your loved one or friend out of the facility for a meal from time to time and/or bring them food that you know they are particularly fond of.

9

DIRECT CARE NEEDS

Dissatisfaction with the care a resident receives will more than likely account for at least 80% of the conflict you may experience while in a nursing home. Some aspects of direct care needs are outlined below and the potential problems that are, from time to time, likely to occur. I will expand on such direct care needs as clothing/dressing, toileting, incontinence, dentures and oral care, glasses, hearing aids, hygiene and grooming, meals/feeding, and naps.

As a resident is a nursing home, you may be independent with your dressing needs, or you may require supervision, limited assistance, extensive assistance, or you may be totally dependent on direct care staff for your dressing needs. Medical conditions that influence your level of care as it relates to your dressing needs may include tremors of the extremities related to Parkinson's disease, partial or full paralysis of your extremities related to a stroke (also known as a CVA), arthritis that makes it difficult to manipulate buttons or snaps, visual deficits that make it difficult to line up buttons or snaps and difficulty matching clothing colors, etc.

A resident's inability to adequately meet their dressing needs may be influenced by a diagnosis of dementia that affects a resident's cognitive status as it relates their dressing needs. Residents with dementia may still be able to recognize clothing as their own but cannot recall how to put on clothing and in what order such as putting on a pair of slacks and then putting their underwear on over their slacks. They may also put on a blouse, sweater, and/or brassiere backwards, as well as, putting on multiple layers of clothing.

When meals are served, some residents in nursing homes that require assistance with feeding may not permit a staff member to assist. For whatever reason, a resident may not be the neatest eater and the next thing you know, there is a trail of food from the top to the bottom of the resident's shirt or blouse. I have found this usually occurs because a resident is having a great deal of difficulty manipulating eating utensils related to dementia or arthritis, and therefore, food spills off the utensils onto themselves or the floor. If a resident is having difficulty manipulating eating utensils, meet with the dietary supervisor and inquire as to the use of adaptive eating utensils.

If you are a visiting family member and you observe this, your first reaction may be one of serious concern. Regardless of whether a resident is a neat eater or not, if they are making attempts to feed themselves, they should be encouraged to do so to foster independence and it is the responsibility of the direct care staff to assist the resident with grooming and changing into a clean outfit when the resident has completed their meal.

Where the problem often lies and contributes to conflicts between a resident, family members, and staff is when a resident is wandering around the nursing home for three to four hours after they have completed their meal, and are oblivious to the fact that their clothes are as stained as they are. This is where it is very important that staff, and I mean all staff members in a nursing home, are observant and motivated in ensuring that, as soon as possible after a meal, a resident is cleaned and changed if they are observed wearing stained clothing. It is a matter of protecting and ensuring a resident's dignity.

As a family member, you may have been told that a resident's clothes are stained because they just completed their lunch meal, when in fact the resident completed their lunch meal one to three hours ago. As a resident or family member of a resident and this becomes a common occurrence, meet with the nurse manager and request that a different caregiver be assigned to you or your family member during meal times.

There are residents in nursing homes that are continent of bowel and bladder, may have occasional episodes of bowel or bladder incontinence, or are totally incontinent of bowel and bladder. Residents that are continent of bowel and bladder, toileting themselves is a relatively easy task unless they have physical deficits that require the physical assistance of staff. Residents that experience occasional episodes of bowel and bladder should be encouraged to toilet themselves, if able, every two to three hours to hopefully avoid the embarrassment that often accompanies an episode of incontinence. A resident who is occasionally incontinent of bladder may want to consider wearing liners in their undergarments in the event they experience a minor episode of incontinence.

A great number of residents in nursing homes are cognitively impaired and cannot follow a bowel and bladder program that encourages them to toilet themselves every two to three hours. Incontinent residents that are cognitively impaired are dependent on staff to provide the toileting assistance they require to hopefully be free from episodes of incontinence.

If you are a resident in a nursing home, or a family member of a resident who is occasionally incontinent, whether it bowel, bladder, or both, meet with the nurse manager and request that incontinent briefs not be used. The staff should be teaching and encouraging residents to toilet themselves regularly or assisting a resident with toileting. Once in a while, you will find a staff member who insists on using incontinence briefs on a resident who is occasionally incontinent because they may feel they do not have the time to encourage a resident to toilet themselves every two to three hours. The longer a resident remains in a soiled brief, the higher the risk of skin breakdown.

For all incontinent residents in a nursing home who are planning to leave the facility for any extended period of time, the direct care staff should ensure that a resident is toileted prior to leaving the nursing home and upon returning to the nursing home. Having an episode of incontinence while out of the nursing home can be quite embarrassing for a resident and their family. As a family member who plans on taking their loved one out of a nursing home at times, you should learn how to change an incontinence brief and if you do not have one with you, request one from the nursing home.

As a general rule, incontinent residents should be checked, cleaned, and changed as needed every two to three hours while awake, when they awaken in the morning, before and after meals, prior to attending structured activities, prior to and upon returning to the nursing home, before going to bed at night, and at the same time intervals during the night while they are sleeping.

If, as a resident or a family member of a resident in a nursing home, you observe incontinence briefs used when they should not be or the staff is double-briefing, meet with the nurse manager to hopefully ensure that this matter is quickly corrected. If you are not pleased with the nurse manager's response or inaction, meet with the Director of Nursing and the Administrator. Double-briefing is another reason why you should closely scrutinize your monthly billing statement because you may be paying for quite a bit more incontinence briefs than necessary.

Another issue related to resident care in a nursing home is providing adequate oral care and denture cleaning to residents that require this assistance. Many residents in nursing homes are cognitively able to manage their oral care or denture needs, however, a great number of residents are cognitively impaired and are no longer able to brush their teeth independently or able to manage their dentures as it relates to daily cleaning or storing their dentures properly and must rely on staff to manage this very important health care need for them.

A common complaint I have heard from visitors and family members when visiting is that a resident had food "caked" in their teeth or a resident's dentures were "floating" around in their mouth because the staff did not use denture adhesive or the dentures do not fit properly. Residents should have proper oral care upon awakening, after meals, prior to going to bed, and as needed. Should you as a friend/family member of a resident in a nursing home observe that they have food particles in their teeth or dentures are not put in or are not fitted properly, immediately meet with the assigned nurse or nurse manager to share your concerns.

As a resident or a family member, you may become livid when you are informed that your/their dentures are missing. The only thing you can think of at the moment is how is a resident going to eat without their dentures, how much is it going to cost to replace the dentures, and who is going to absorb this cost.

Although most nursing homes have measures in place to hopefully ensure that dentures do not become lost such as placing then in a secure and designated place, in a proper denture container, and clearly marked with the resident's name. Family members of residents that are cognitively impaired must realize that their loved one may very well take their dentures out themselves and place them anywhere such as wrapped up in a napkin on their meal tray and they become discarded along with the contents of the meal tray. Dentures get wrapped up in a resident's bed linens and sub-sequently are sent to the laundry or you may have a cognitively impaired roommate who has taken your dentures and put them who knows where. When lost dentures are found, it is very difficult to assess what resident they belong too. Having dentures engraved with a resident's name or initials is very helpful when missing dentures are located. When a resident is missing their dentures and must now move about the nursing home without their dentures, it becomes a serious dignity issue.

Keeping track of residents' glasses in nursing homes is just as difficult as keeping track of dentures. A great deal of residents in nursing homes have visual deficits and must rely on their glasses to be able to read, attend structured activities, and to navigate the nursing home. Many residents take off their glasses and leave them in various areas of the nursing home. Some staff members are observant as to a resident's style of glasses and are able to identify the owner when glasses are found. Many family members reside out of the area and are not available to identify their loved ones missing glasses. Cognitively impaired residents are usually unable to identify their own glasses when they are found. Just as one can have dentures engraved with their name or initials, one can also have their glasses engraved in the event they become lost and are later found.

For quite a few residents in nursing homes, hearing aids are essentially their lifeline as it relates to being able to communicate with others who share their environment. Just like dentures and glasses, cognitively impaired residents often misplace their hearing aids and/or do not recall how to properly care for and store their hearing aids. How about the cognitively impaired resident who places their hearing aids in their denture cup thinking that it is the case to store their hearing aids, and yes, the denture cup is full of water? Not good for the resident or the hearing aids.

Just as lost dentures and glasses have a negative impact on a resident's functional status within the nursing home, lost hearing aids impacts the staff's ability to effectively communicate with a resident during care. While some facilities are diligent enough to ensure that residents' dentures, glasses, and hearing aids are stored in a safe place when not in use such as when a resident is being bathed or is in bed for the night, you can bet that, from time to time, dentures, glasses, and hearing aids will turn up missing, especially on a dementia or Alzheimer's unit.

Hearing aids can also be engraved with a resident's initials so that it is easier to identify to whom they belong when missing hearing aids are located. Some residents and family members become so frustrated when hearing aids become missing, they have resorted to leasing hearing aids that are insured and will likely be replaced when lost or damaged. Once again, during the admissions process, it is very important to inquire as to whom is responsible for replacing lost dentures, glasses, and hearing aids, you or the nursing home. This can be a real tricky area because it can be very difficult to assess whether dentures, glasses, or hearing aides are missing due to staff negligence versus a resident misplacing them themselves.

If you as health care surrogate and/or power of attorney for a cognitively impaired resident in a nursing home, meet with the nurse manager and insist that your loved ones dentures, glasses, and hearing aids are locked in a safe place by staff every day. Taking this approach, should they become missing, you should put up your best defense that the nursing home be held responsible for replacing the lost items. I use the word "defense" because a nursing home is not going to be pleased about replacing the lost items because they can be quite costly.

Hygiene and grooming needs can be a challenge for residents in nursing homes that are cognitively intact related to medical issues or physical deficits and cognitively impaired residents are certain to require some level of assistance with their hygiene and grooming needs.

Many residents in nursing homes leave the facility from time to time for medical appointments or they are planning to spend the day with friends and family members. As a family member planning to take a resident out of the facility for whatever reason, you may become somewhat livid when you arrive at the nursing home only to find your loved still dressed in their pajamas, possibly unshaven and not groomed, even though you gave staff explicit instructions that you would pick up the resident at a certain time. As a family member who is unaware as to the daily functioning of a nursing home, hopefully after you read this book, you will find that it more practical to arrive at the nursing home at a time that will permit a little time cushion. Getting residents up for the day can be a long, tedious process and there is a wide range of variables that can influence care issues being completed on a timely basis, therefore, do not come down to hard on the staff when your loved one is not ready to leave the nursing home at a certain time.

It is also very important to not be late when picking up a resident for a visit outside the facility, as while they are awaiting your arrival, they may have an episode of incontinence that will now require more time to ensure that the resident is clean and dry when they leave the nursing home. As a resident or a family member, should you feel that hygiene and grooming needs are not being met, be sure to meet with your nurse manager.

Residents in nursing homes often become fatigued quite easily, especially if they are very active in structured activities offered by the nursing home. They often require brief naps to regain the energy they require to continue to pursue activities of interest. Family members often become angry and frustrated when they arrive for a visit to find their loved one exhausted, especially when they were planning on taking their loved one out of the facility for a while. Some staff members are reluctant at times to assist a resident in getting in bed for a nap because it may be meal time in an hour or so and they do not want to have to get the resident out of bed for their meal.

How often have you visited a nursing home only to find some residents sleeping in their wheelchairs in common areas of the nursing home? This generally occurs for one of two reasons. A resident may be exhausted and/or there is not enough social stimulation to ensure a resident is awake while in common areas of the nursing home. Residents who are unable to self-propel their wheelchairs may have been placed where they are by staff and the staff member then left the resident there by themselves. I have often heard family members demand that their loved one have a nap starting at a set time everyday. This may be somewhat unrealistic depending on what else is going on in the nursing home at the time, and other residents care needs may have priority over their loved one being laid down for nap at a set time everyday. Try to be somewhat flexible.

10

DISCHARGE PLANNING

Discharge planning is such a vital service provided by a nursing home and practically commences upon admission to a nursing home. The social worker in a nursing home is generally responsible for discharge planning however a resident's physician or ARNP must write a discharge order prior to a resident being discharged from a nursing home.

Some residents that are admitted to nursing homes are admitted on a permanent basis from the very start. Others are planning to enter a nursing home for hopefully a short period of time such as requiring short term rehabilitation for a knee or hip replacement, as a respite (break) for their in-home caregiver and/or family members, or the family may be traveling and cannot take their loved one with them.

Discharge planning generally does not involve residents that are admitted to a nursing home on a permanent basis unless they were to improve significantly and reassessed as to the possibility of being able to reside in a lesser restrictive environment such as home, residing with a family member, or relocating to an assisted living facility. There will also be quite a bit of discharge planning should a resident be issued a thirty day notice of transfer/discharge from a nursing home.

For residents that are more than likely to be short term admissions, there is quite a bit of discharge planning involved. The social worker must consult with the physician, the ARNP, the Care Plan Team, and the nursing staff to assess the prognosis of a resident being able to return home or their former residence.

The social worker must meet with family members to discuss a resident's medical and/or cognitive status to assess whether their caregiver, family, spouse, or friend are going to be able to meet the resident's care needs at home, with or without in-home health care services and durable medical equipment such as a walker, wheelchair, hospital bed, high top commode, and grab bars in the tub or shower to name a few. This is exactly why a short term resident and/or their family should attend a resident's initial Care Plan Conference. Remember, this conference is where a resident and family will learn about a residents care needs and what level of progress a resident must attain before they may be able to return home or to their former residence. Should a resident not meet their goals in therapy, and/or cannot be cared for at home by their family, they may become a permanent resident in a nursing home. When this occurs, a resident and their family may experience emotional difficulties (see the chapter on mental health issues).

I have observed many a resident in a nursing home that because of their anger, frustration, and/or depression related to their placement in a nursing home, they were very unco-operative with therapy and rather than progress in therapy, they regressed in therapy and very well may have jeopardized their chances of returning home. I have met some very patient physical, occupational, and speech therapists how-ever if a resident continually refuses to cooperate in therapy, they are going to be discharged from therapy in a relatively short period of time and may also jeopardize their Medicare benefits in the nursing home.

Therefore, as a resident in a nursing home, if it is your desire to be able to return home, I strongly suggest that you do your best to cooperate with your assigned therapists. If anger and/or depression is a issue, you can receive mental health services while in the nursing home for a short period of time. It is also generally the responsibility of the social worker to order in-home durable medical equipment for a resident being discharged from a nursing home. The social worker will also arrange any needed in-home health care ser-vices such as physical, occupational, or speech therapy, oxy-gen, an in-home caregiver for bathing, and grooming/hygiene needs, or a meals-on-wheels program. The social worker may also arrange in-home hospice care for residents that are terminally ill, as well as, pastoral services.

11

FUNERAL ARRANGEMENTS

The number of residents in their 70's, 80's, and 90's who have not made funeral arrangements may surprise you. When people have attained these ages, I cannot help but think that, from time to time, they have thought about what will happen to their possessions and remains upon death. For some individuals, the thought of making funeral arrangements are a reminder of our mortality and cannot bring themselves to make their funeral arrangements.

Residents and family members of residents who have not made funeral arrangements may not be able to fully appreciate the impact this has on family members and a nursing home when a resident passes away. Most nursing homes do not have the accommodations to store a corpse therefore they are often at a loss as to what to do with a corpse until arrangements are made with a funeral home or cremation service. If funeral arrangements are not made prior to passing away, a nursing home must relocate the deceased resident's roommate if they have one until the deceased is picked up by a funeral home or a cremation service.

Often, family members reside out of state and are not familiar with funeral homes in the local area. When a resident without funeral arrangements passes away, generally, it is the responsibility of the social worker to contact the family and furnish them the names and phone numbers of local nursing homes or cremation services so the family can make arrangements and compare costs associated with making funeral arrangements.

When a resident passes away without funeral arrangements and the family cannot be reached, the deceased must often remain in the nursing home for extended periods of time. If to much time has elapsed, the social worker may have to contact local funeral homes to assess whether they are willing to pick up the deceased until family can be contacted and referred to the funeral home.

As a resident or a family member of a resident in a nursing home, do your best to ensure that funeral arrangements are made as soon as possible after admission to the nursing home so that your family does not find themselves in a panic and having to disrupt their lives and scramble at the last minute making funeral arrangements. Be sure to address this issue during the admissions process.

12

HEALTH INFORMATION PORTABILITY ACCOUNTABILITY ACT (HIPAA)

This act became effective on April 14, 2003 and relates to when and how your health information may be shared with others. As a resident or a health care decision maker for someone in a nursing home, it is very important for you to be aware of how and when information about your medical status, medical history, diagnosis/prognosis, and medical records may be released to others.

As a resident in a hospital, nursing home, assisted living facility, or receiving outpatient medical services, you have certain rights as to how and when your medical information may be shared with others. You can: 1) restrict certain uses and disclosures of your medical information; 2) inspect and request copies of your medical records but it may involve paying a fee to the health care provider; 3) revoke authorization to disclose your health care information by request at any time.

While you may have to pay a fee for copies of your medical records, it is very important that you obtain copies of your medical records because trying to recall when and the type of medical care you received in the past, can be quite difficult for most individuals. Also be sure to request copies of the Notice of Privacy Practices from all of your health care providers.

Long before this act was put into effect, all nursing homes had to conform to a strict policy as it related to confidentially of residents medical information. As a social worker in a nursing home, on many occasions, I had to meet with angry family members because they were not, in writing, authorized to receive medical information about their family member in the nursing home. I can appreciate the frustration that a family member may feel when denied access to their family member's medical information however laws are laws. As a family member or a health care surrogate, getting angry, demanding, or being verbally abusive to the staff is not going to solve this issue. As a family member, should this occur, request to meet with the social worker to assess what can be done, or what cannot be done, for you to be able to receive information related to your loved ones medical status.

I can also fully appreciate an individual's medical information being kept confidential per their request. Family members do not always have a caring, loving relationship, therefore, it is a resident's right to choose what information, if any, can be shared with a particular family member. A resident's right to confidentiality also extends to outside agencies.

If a resident in a nursing home lacks capacity to make their own health care decisions, their appointed health care surrogate, proxy, or legal guardian has the right to determine who will be authorized to receive medical information concerning the resident. Sometimes there is quite a bit of discord between family members and when a health care decision maker denies another family member authorization to receive medical information related to their family member in a nursing home, it usually has a negative impact on the resident, the family, and the nursing home.

As a resident with capacity, a health care surrogate, proxy, or legal guardian, upon admission to a nursing home, request to sign release of information forms to determine who is authorized to receive medical information about a resident. For the nursing home, this will greatly reduce confusion as to who is authorized to receive medical information about a resident and also hopefully prevent medical information from being released to unauthorized individuals and agencies. When this occurs, it is a serious breach of resident's rights.

Many employees in nursing homes have been terminated because they released information regarding a resident without proper authorization. They may have meant well but were either uninformed as to who is authorized to receive information about a resident or they may have felt intimidated by an angry, demanding, family member to disclose a resident's medical information. Family members must realize that staff members in nursing homes must follow the law and it is the family's responsibility to deal with and attempt to resolve any discord there may be amongst family members.

13

HOPE/HOSPICE SERVICES

I am not going to go into great depth about hope/hospice services as one can contact their local hope/hospice organization and request one of their manuals that outline their mission, criteria for admission, and the services they provide.

As it relates to residents in nursing homes, should a resident physically and/or cognitively deteriorate to the point where a resident's primary physician feels it is their medical judgment that the resident is now terminally ill, the physician will write an order for a resident to be referred to Hope/Hospice pending a resident's authorization if they have capacity, or that of a health care surrogate, proxy, or legal guardian. A rule of thumb some physicians follow related to a diagnosis of terminal illness is whether their medical opinion is such that they feel a resident may have less than six months of life expectancy. Should this be the case, once an order is written for the referral and a release of information is secured, generally the nurse manager or the social worker will contact hope/hospice with basic referral information and hope/hospice staff will come to the nursing home and conduct an evaluation to assess whether a resident's medical condition meets Hospice admission criteria.

As a family member or an appointed health care decision maker, do not panic should you receive a call requesting a referral to Hope/Hospice. This does not necessarily mean that your loved one is on death's doorstep. You should request that a Care Plan conference be scheduled prior to agreeing to a referral or admission to Hope/Hospice. Prior to meeting with the care plan team, request to meet with the resident's physician to assess why they feel a referral to Hope/Hospice is indicated. Also request that a representative from Hope/Hospice attend the Care Plan conference. On a positive note, residents in nursing homes can generally receive hospice services in the nursing home, however, a resident or their appointed health care decision maker can request that a resident be relocated to an inpatient hospice facility.

When the time is appropriate to possibly relocate to an inpatient hospice facility, be sure to inquire as to the financial impact the relocation may have on you, if any, versus continuing to receive hospice services while residing in a nursing home of your choice. Be sure to inquire as to what your Medicare and/or Medicaid benefits will cover while receiving the services of Hope/Hospice.

14

HOUSEKEEPING SERVICES

Housekeeping services provided by a nursing home can certainly be a challenge for the staff, residents, and their families. It is not a very glamorous job and thank God there are people willing to work in this capacity. Spending most of the work day cleaning numerous rooms, moping up spills such as food, vomit, urine, and feces, and disposing of numerous bags containing soiled incontinence supplies can be difficult at times. Some residents in nursing homes are not the tidiest individuals and generally have a habit of throwing tissues, newspapers, etc. on the floor, as opposed to, placing them in the trash receptacle.

Often, housekeeping staff clean a room, only to have to return in a short period of time because a cognitively impaired resident managed to turn the room into a disaster rather quickly. Some residents are constantly moving things around in their room and when family members visit, they are often aghast as to how untidy or disorganized the room is.

At times, family members have a great deal of difficulty accepting that their loved one could make such a mess of their room because they share that "all their life, they were such a neat and tidy person". When a resident's room looks like a disaster, family members and visitors are sometimes too quick to criticize the housekeeping staff, not realizing that they may not necessarily be responsible for the appearance of a room.

Most housekeeping staff members are very conscientious employees who strive to do their best as it relates to ensuring that a nursing home is as clean as possible and there are others that exhibit performance that only meets minimum standards. Housekeeping staff should be closely monitored to ensure that they are on top of things as it relates to cleanliness as I cannot stress the importance of cleanliness in a nursing home enough.

Due to a nursing home being a communal living environment, at times, it is very difficult to contain certain germs, viruses, etc., and therefore, residents may be at risk of contracting various forms of ailments. This can occur in the cleanest of nursing homes, however, nursing homes that do not provide adequate housekeeping services only increase the risk of residents becoming ill.

As a nursing home, ensure that spills of any sort within your facility are given priority over some other housekeeping tasks in the event a resident, family member, visitor, or staff member experiences a fall with injuries that may potentially invite a lawsuit against the nursing home. As a resident, family member, or visitor in a nursing home, before you become to quick to criticize and possibly belittle the housekeeping staff, consider some of the examples mentioned above that contribute to the disarray that may occur from time to time, however, if cleanliness appears to be a chronic problem, be sure to meet with the housekeeping supervisor to hopefully resolve this problem.

15

LAUNDRY

As a resident being admitted to a nursing home, you may request that the nursing home do your laundry on a regular basis and hopefully be reassured that you will always have clean clothes on a daily basis, your laundry will not turn up missing, and your laundry will be returned to you as promptly as possible. Think again.

Picture this. Not long after being admitted to the nursing home, you are looking for that special outfit you had planned to wear for the day and/or for a special event you planned on attending. You look high and low to no avail. By now, you may start to panic and start to wonder "what am I going to do now?"

A staff member comes to your room and informs you that your outfit cannot be located. By this time, your pulse is racing and the tops of your ears are bright red, not to mention what this is doing to your blood pressure. Your main concern at this point is what more is going to done to locate your outfit, and if not found, is the nursing home financially liable for replacing your outfit.

During the admissions process, be sure to inquire about having a resident's clothing labeled with their name so that hopefully their clothes will return to their room. Be sure to inquire as to whether there is a charge for this service. If, as a family member, you prefer to label your loved one's clothes yourself, please label them on the inside and not the outside of the clothes as this is considered a dignity issue. You may consider this common sense however, over the years I have observed residents in nursing homes wandering the facility with their name on the outside in big, bold, black magic marker.

Should your clothes get lost, meet with the supervisor of the laundry department and discuss your dissatisfaction. They will generally reassure you that everything is being done to locate your outfit and assure you that future service will be to your satisfaction. At this point, you may feel confident that this issue is resolved and you can expect satisfactory service in the future.

Several weeks go by and once again your number one outfit is missing or you have no socks, pants, shirts, blouses, bras, etc. You meet, once again, with the supervisor of the laundry department to share your concerns only to hear that the laundry service will improve, however it will certainly happen again. All you can hope for at this point is that this does not become a chronic problem.

Just as the kitchen churns out hundreds of meals a day, the laundry department does their best to ensure that copious amounts of laundry are cleaned and delivered to residents rooms on a daily basis. Labels come off. Clothes labels made in magic marker wear off. Where do you think this laundry ends up? In the corner of the laundry room where clothes are piled up that cannot be identified. For a staff member looking for a lost outfit, this could be like looking for a needle in a haystack.

Nursing homes must ensure that employees in the laundry department are able to read residents name labels. I mention this because clothes often end up in the wrong rooms and the general consensus may be that some staff members have difficulty reading or comprehending residents' names. When residents and family members become so frustrated and feel at the end their rope as it relates to missing laundry, they are often perplexed as to what to do to rectify this situation. They may have lost confidence in the services provided by the laundry department.

One solution is to inquire as to whether there are employees within the nursing home who will launder a resident's clothes on a private pay basis. Often, this improves your odds of your clothes being laundered on a regular basis, minimizes the chances of missing clothes, and hopefully, you will always have that special outfit available to you.

When negotiating with a staff member to do your laundry on a private pay basis, it is very important to remember that if you have any complaints about the staff member doing your laundry, you cannot expect the nursing home to become involved because you chose to make laundry arrangements on your own. If you hire an independent person to do your laundry, the nursing home is no longer responsible for missing and/or damaged laundry. When negotiating with a staff member or independent individual to do your laundry on a private pay basis while in a nursing home, be sure to obtain in writing how often the laundry will be picked up, the turn around time for the laundry to be returned, and who is responsible for replacing damaged or lost clothing.

When negotiating with an individual to do your laundry, a good rule of thumb related to how much to pay this individual is to not pay any more than the nursing home charges to do your laundry. I have found that residents and family members are generally more satisfied with hiring private pay individuals to do their laundry than entrusting a nursing home with doing their laundry.

Laundry issues on a dementia unit is further complicated because often, residents that are diagnosed with dementia, often go "shopping" where they routinely take clothes belonging to others residents and either wear the clothes that do not belong to them, or they relocate other residents clothing to various areas of the nursing home. When this occurs, it usually infuriates family members. If the clothes are clearly labeled, the odds of them returning to the rightful owner are fairly good, however, on quite a few occasions, missing clothes are never recovered.

Because of the issue of missing clothes on a dementia unit, a common sense approach for residents and family members is to purchase inexpensive clothes for residents to wear on a daily basis that are clearly labeled with the resident's name, usually on the inside of the collar, and bring any "special" outfits from home for the resident to wear the day they are planning to attend a special event and be sure to take the outfit home with you at the end of the day.

16

LIFE CARE COMMUNITIES

Many older folks are not knowledgeable regarding the concept of life care communities which generally offer independent living services, assisted living services, and skilled nursing services all on the same campus and generally have minimum age requirements so be sure to inquire about this when assessing life care communities.

A life care community generally sells an apartment to an aged individual or couple and they are charged a monthly maintenance fee that is usually based on the particular apartment that was sold, as well as, the square footage of the apartment. The amount of the monthly maintenance fee may change from time depending on budgetary issues and the rising cost of living. The monthly maintenance fee generally includes some costs associated with having to enter the nursing home of the life care community.

Residents in life care communities generally start out in an independent apartment. As time passes and a resident starts to deteriorate physically and/or cognitively to the point where they can no longer function in their apartment independently, they usually relocate to the communities assisted living facility and generally pay the same or close to the same monthly maintenance fee they were paying in their independent apartment and will now receive the assisted living services they require. PRIOR to relocating to an assisted living apartment, inquire as to what the effect this may have on your monthly maintenance fee if any. Also inquire as to how the monthly maintenance fee is impacted should only one of the couple require relocation to assisted living while their mate remains in their independent apartment.

Should a resident in the assisted living part of a life care community deteriorate even further, and it is determined by their assigned physician that their care needs can longer be met in an assisted living environment, they will be requested or made to relocate to the communities skilled care nursing home.

A major benefit of some life care communities is a resident may be admitted to their skilled nursing home as often as they require such placement and generally are not charged a per diem rate for daily services provided by the nursing home whereas a private pay resident from outside of the life care community would be charged a hefty per diem rate for services they received while in the nursing home. Keep in mind that your monthly maintenance fee may only cover room and board while in the nursing home. As a resident of the life care community nursing home, you may be responsible for payment of services provided by the nursing home such as, laundry, telephone, medications, medical supplies, as well as, other fees. Be sure to inquire as to what your financial responsibility is should you require placement in the nursing home of the life care community.

While investigating life care communities for possible relocation, be sure to meet with the sales department and inquire as to ALL of your financial obligations regardless whether you reside in your independent apartment, their assisted living facility, or their skilled nursing home. While making these inquiries, remember that all services provided by the life care community are made on a contractual basis and may become quite complex and confusing, therefore, be sure you understand all entities in the contract prior to sign-ing any documents. You may very well want to acquire the services of a real estate attorney to provide guidance during the complex negotiations. Know exactly what services you can expect for payment rendered.

When meeting with a sales person from a life care com-munity, also be sure to inquire as to other services offered by the life care community such as housekeeping services in your apartment, transportation to medical appointments, grocery stores, malls, etc. Be sure to inquire as to various structured activities offered by a life care community to assess whether the activities offered are compatible with activity interests that you generally enjoy.

Some life care communities may be affiliated with a particular religion. If you are considering relocating to a life care community that is affiliated with a particular religion be as sure as you can that your religious/spiritual beliefs do not conflict with the religious/spiritual beliefs of the life care community. You do not have to convert to the communities religious affiliation, however, if there is a major conflict related to religious preferences, you may find yourself quite unhappy residing in the life care community. Inquire about the rules and possible restrictions implemented by the life care community. For example, a life care community that is affiliated with a particular religion may prohibit consuming alcoholic beverages in their dining rooms or restaurants. They may also ban dancing in public places within the life care community. If you enjoy an alcoholic beverage while dining out and/or enjoy dancing, a life care community that is affiliated with a particular religion may not be for you. Also, be sure to inquire as to the communities' policy related to allowing relatives, friends, etc. to reside in your apartment for brief or extended time periods whether you are home or not.

What I consider to be a very negative aspect of residing in a life care community is they more than likely have a policy that you may never re-sell your independent apartment and should you have to relocate to assisted living or the skilled nursing home on a permanent basis, the life care community may regain ownership of your independent apartment for resale purposes. Given this thought, should you find yourself becoming very disenchanted with life in a life care community, you may be stuck because you cannot sell your independent apartment and you may need the equity you have in the apartment to relocate to a more suitable community. Should a resident or couple become so unhappy residing in their life care community, they can meet with administrators to discuss their discontent and hopefully a compromise can be reached where a buyout of your contract may be proposed. Whether a life care community is affiliated with a particular religion or not, you can bet they want to get their hands on every dollar they can and may offer you a buyout of your contract that you find insufficient and/or insulting.

The bottom line is, be sure to do your homework when it comes to considering possible relocation to a life care community because if you are unsuccessful having your contract amended or nullified, you have essentially two choices; remain in the life care community and be miserable, or leave and lose whatever equity you had in your apartment.

17

MEDICAL CONSULTANTS

As a resident in a nursing home, you will more than likely require the services of numerous medical consultants such as a primary physician, podiatrist, dentist, optometrist, neurologist, audiologist, psychiatrist, psychologist, urologist, oncologist, gastroenterologist, dermatologist, orthopedic and cardiac specialists, and more. Keeping track of all your medical consultants can be quite a challenge.

As a resident, you will more than likely have numerous concerns as to how to manage multiple medical appointments. Do not worry. Your treating physician or ARNP will write orders for the medical appointments that are required related to your medical needs and the unit secretary is generally responsible for making your medical appointments with the appropriate health care providers and will also assist with making transportation arrangements to your appointment should you have difficulty arranging transportation on your own. As a resident, you can also schedule your own medical appointments. If you do, be sure to inform the nursing staff and the unit secretary so they are aware you will be out of the facility.

Depending on your medical status, cognitive status, and functional disabilities, you may require the services of a non-emergency transportation company to transport you to your medical appointments. Also, depending on your medical and/or cognitive status, you may also need to be accompanied to your appointment by a private duty aide who can attend to your needs while at your medical appointment, and you will more than likely be responsible for the charges incurred.

If you are a Medicaid recipient in a nursing home, your selection of non-emergency transportation providers may be limited to certain transportation providers, therefore, as a Medicaid recipient in a nursing home, be sure to inform the unit secretary of this so that they can ensure that the proper transportation provider is contacted. Do not assume that all unit secretaries are aware of the payment status of the residents in a nursing home.

As a Medicaid recipient and the incorrect transportation provider was scheduled by the staff, should you receive a bill for the charges, meet with the Administrator of the nursing home as soon as possible and insist that the nursing home assume responsibility for the transportation charges. If the Administrator refuses to assume payment for the transportation charges, contact your Ombudsman's Council who oversees resident's rights in nursing homes and request their intervention (see chapter related to the Ombudsman's Council).

If your medical status is not considered serious or fragile, your physician may authorize a family member or a friend to transport you to your medical appointments as this would be sure to save you quite a bit of money by not having to pay for non-emergency transportation charges. As a resident in a nursing home without family or friends in the local area to assist with your transportation needs, meet with the social worker in the nursing home and inquire as to whether there are volunteer drivers or organizations that can assist you with transportation to your medical appointments.

18

MEDICARE AND MEDICAID BENEFITS

Comprehending Medicare and Medicaid regulations can certainly be a challenge for most folks. With Medicare and Medicaid guidelines/criteria changing from time to time, one must be quite astute to be able to keep up with the changes. Because the guidelines do change, it is my intention to give you an overview of basic Medicare and Medicaid guidelines. An individual who is eligible for Medicare and Medicaid must realize that Medicare and Medicaid guidelines differ as it relates to outpatient care, hospitalization, and nursing home placement.

Certain criteria must be met before a resident can be admitted to a nursing home under Medicare guidelines. A general requirement may be that a person must spend at least three days in a general hospital. Discharge planning at the hospital should include assessing whether it may be appropriate for you to be admitted to a skilled nursing home for a short period of time for physical and/or occupational therapy secondary to a knee or hip replacement or physical deficits related to a stroke or other medical issues requiring nursing home placement. If you are admitted to a nursing home, in a very short period of time, you should be assessed by the nursing, therapy, dietary, and social services department. Upon admission to a nursing home, it is very important to inquire as to your Medicare/Medicaid benefits while in the nursing home and also request copies of your benefits.

Should you no longer require skilled therapy and/or skilled nursing services, you will more than likely be decertified from Medicare. A decision now has to be made whether you are well enough to return home or do you continue to require inpatient care in the nursing home. Should you require further care in the nursing home, you will more than likely convert to private pay status unless you qualify for Medicaid benefits or have long term care insurance.

Another very important thing to remember as a resident in a nursing home under Medicare A is you are not permitted to leave the nursing home grounds except to attend medical appointments. I believe the logic here from a Medicare perspective is that if you are well enough to go out to dinner, visiting family and friends, and shopping, you may not continue to require nursing home placement.

If your physician or ARNP feels that you are medically stable, request that an order be written for a three to four hour "therapeutic outing" that would afford you quality time with your family and friends outside of the institutional setting of the nursing home. As a resident who is requesting a therapeutic outing, it would not hurt at this point to share that a therapeutic leave may be just what you need to get "rid of the blues".

You cannot request an overnight therapeutic outing while under Medicare A guidelines in a nursing home. As a resident, be careful you do not request therapeutic outings to often as the nursing home may feel that you are abusing this wonderful opportunity and also limit your requests to three to four hours. You will have more success with this approach.

While some residents in nursing homes have attained maximum benefit from therapy, they may not have attained a level of independence sufficient enough to return home or to an assisted living facility as it relates to what is referred to activities of daily living that includes care related to bathing, dressing, eating, toileting, etc.

If you are a resident in a nursing home as described above, be sure to meet with your care plan team to assess whether you may be able to return home if you were able to employ in-home assistance with your activities of daily living. If you are fortunate to be able to go home, also inquire if there are Medicare benefits you may be eligible to receive for in-home care.

If you do not have the financial resources to employ in-home health care assistance and your treating physician feels that you require continued nursing home placement, you are more than likely to become a permanent resident of the nursing home. This will certainly be a difficult time in your life and you will require ongoing emotional support to adjust to placement.

Now that Medicare is no longer paying your nursing home bills and you have very limited financial resources, you may find yourself starting to panic and feel that the nursing home may "put me out on the street". This is not going to happen to you. While you may feel some pressure from the accounting department or the Administrator of the nursing home as it relates to payment for services rendered, simply inform the accounting department and the Administrator that you plan on meeting with the social worker for assistance with applying for Medicaid. Do not permit the representatives of the accounting department or the Administrator of a nursing home to intimidate you as it relates to payment status.

While applying for Medicaid services, you will continue to receive monthly billing statements from the accounting department. If you are approved to receive Medicaid, reimbursement is generally paid to the nursing on a retroactive basis to the date you applied for Medicaid. It may be easier to convert to Medicaid while already in a nursing home than being admitted to a nursing home under Medicaid from the beginning. Nursing homes generally structure budgets to account for a certain number of private pay, Medicare, and Medicaid beds, if they accept Medicaid at all.

The lesson to learn here is if you are in a nursing home under Medicare A, you know that you cannot afford private pay status, and your prognosis for being able to return home is quite slim, meet with the social worker and initiate the Medicaid process. Your Medicaid application can take up to ninety days to process.

I have heard countless stories from admissions representatives that a resident or family member swore they had enough money to pay for at least six months of care as a private pay resident only to apply for Medicaid one month after admission to the nursing home. It is very important as a resident or family member who is placing a resident in a nursing home to be as honest as possible with the admissions coordinator as it relates to financial resources because it minimizes conflict and you should want to start off "on the right foot" with the nursing home right from the beginning. To be dishonest with the admissions coordinator only jeopardizes trust. On the other hand, do not be too quick to mention Medicaid when meeting with an Admissions Coordinator because they may feel that you will apply for Medicaid shortly after admission.

If as a resident or family member of a resident in a nursing home, should you feel that a nursing home is putting too much financial pressure on you while you are in the process of applying/qualifying for Medicaid, contact your local Long Term Care Ombudsman's office.

If as a resident or family member, you are having quite a bit of difficulty qualifying for Medicaid, it will cost you money in the short term and could save you quite a bit of money in the long term, but I would suggest that you seek the services of an Elder Law attorney.

Purchasing long term care insurance and a prescription medication plan can certainly help defray some of the exorbitant costs associated with nursing home placement however, you should purchase long term care insurance well in advance of your need to be admitted to a nursing and when you are more than likely to not have any pre-existing medical conditions.

19

MEDICATION

One thing you will usually find is that some nursing homes generally prefer that new admissions to their facility obtain their medications from a pharmacy of their choice however, as a resident in a nursing home you should have the right to obtain your prescribed medications from a pharmacy of YOUR choice.

Be very cautious of nursing homes that have their own pharmacy and insist that residents obtain their prescribed medications from their pharmacy where the cost of medications may be marked up, ensuring more cost to you and more financial revenue for the nursing home.

Upon admission to a nursing home, inquire as to their policy regarding self-administration of prescribed medications. A nursing home may employ some form of assessment as to whether you are medically and cognitively able to safely administer your own prescribed medications. It you are permitted to self-administer your own medication, it is usually required they be kept in a locked cabinet next to your bedside. This includes all over-the-counter medications also.

When you are reviewing your list of prescribed medications, be sure that any medication or food allergies are on the list and the nursing staff is aware of your medication and food allergies. This is important because some prescription medication is prescribed to be taken with food.

When a nurse administers your medications, inquire as to what each pill, capsule, or liquid is prescribed for and confirm that you are receiving your medications at the prescribed time. Some nurses in nursing homes administer medications when it is convenient for them and not necessarily when they should be administered. This occurs mostly at night when a resident is getting ready for bed and it is easier for the nurse if she gives the resident their nightly medications while they are still awake, as opposed to having to wake a resident up at a later time to administer their medications. The time a medication is prescribed is very important from a medical perspective however some medications may be given an hour before or an hour after the prescribed time. If you observe your nurse administering your medication hours earlier than prescribed, request that they return at the prescribed time and be sure you meet with your nurse manager to share that your nurse is employing this tactic.

All nursing homes are required by law to keep track of when medications are administered. This is done by completing a monthly **Medication Administration Record** referred to as the **MAR**. Every resident in a nursing home must have a new Mar completed every month. The MAR records the medication that is prescribed, the dosage, time of administration, allergies, and any special instructions that may accompany a medication such as whether a medication must be taken with food, or if a resident's blood pressure must be taken prior to the administration of a certain medication.

The MAR also contains any missed does of medication related to resident refusal of medications or they must be destroyed because a medication may have become contaminated for some reason. The bottom line is nurses are only human and from time to time, medication errors do occur. Be sure to keep on top of your prescribed medications as a resident in a nursing home. If you have medication allergies, be sure you wear some form of wristband or Medic Alert bracelet or pendent as to minimize any medical errors and possible medical emergencies.

I probably do not have to tell you about the exorbitant costs associated with prescribed medications, therefore, it would really be to your benefit to purchase prescription medication insurance while you are only prescribed a couple of medications because should you start deteriorating physically, cognitively, and/or behaviorally, the number of your prescribed medications may drastically increase. If you are a resident, a health care surrogate/proxy, or legal guardian of a resident in a nursing home, and are having great difficulty with finances related to your prescribed medications, request a meeting with your treating physician or ARNP to assess whether some medications can be discontinued and/or start shopping around for the most affordable pharmacies because prices pharmacies charge for medications can vary quite a bit and inquire about the use of generic medications as this may save you quite a bit of money.

If you are a health care surrogate/proxy or legal guardian of a resident in a nursing home and the nursing home informs you that your resident refuses medications just about every day, meet with the resident's treating physician or ARNP to assess whether the refused medications can be discontinued. Once a medication is offered to a resident and refused, the medication must be destroyed. You are now paying for medication that is being thrown away.

20

MENTAL HEALTH SERVICES

All nursing homes should contract with mental health providers or offer in-house mental health services to treat residents who are coping with diverse mental health issues that can occur as a result of a resident's medical and/or cognitive status and subsequent need for admission to a nursing home whether it be for a short period of time or permanent basis. Some residents that are diagnosed with some form of dementia exhibit serious mood and/or behavioral deficits at times that must be dealt with and hopefully stabilized.

Given the advanced age of most residents in nursing homes, a great number of residents are diagnosed with serious medical, emotional, and/or cognitive deficits that often leaves residents' experiencing feelings of sadness, anxiety, abandonment, hopelessness, and helplessness. Some residents that lack capacity to make their own health care decisions often feel they have lost all control of their lives because others are now making all of their health care decisions.

A great number of residents I have been fortunate to meet and work for as a social worker have often shared their desire to die at home and always hoped, and sometimes prayed, they would never end up in a nursing home. Now that a resident is in a nursing home, they may have feelings of regret for having lived so long. Often, spouses experience guilt because they promised each other they would never put the other in a nursing home. Promise or not, as a spouse you will more then likely experience feelings of guilt for having to place your spouse in a nursing home. Some elderly folks would prefer to use the term "long term care facility" as opposed to nursing home because they feel there is not as much stigma associated with the term "long term care facility" versus "nursing home".

Depression and anxiety are common psychiatric conditions that often afflict many residents in nursing homes whether they are in a nursing home on a short term basis or a permanent basis. When a resident experiences depression and/or anxiety, they may feel such symptoms as insomnia, helplessness, hopelessness, tearfulness, confusion, agitation, aggression, decreased appetite, lack of motivation to improve, and the loss of pleasure in activities or social circles that used to bring them joy. A resident may begin to refuse care, become resistive or combative with staff, and have a wish to die and/or have thoughts of hastening their own death.

A resident in a nursing home may often minimize their feelings as it relates to mental health issues possibly because of the emotional stigma that unfortunately may still exist today as it relates to being a recipient of mental health services. Having worked with the geriatric population for quite a few years, I recall instances when the mere mention of mental health services would infuriate them and at times would request that I leave. Over the past ten years, I have observed more of an acceptance of mental health services by the geriatric population and many have gone on to lead happy, productive lives.

While it may be somewhat unrealistic for anyone to expect a certified nursing assistant to be knowledgeable of psychiatric symptoms, they can be trained to observe for any changes in their residents demeanor/actions and report their observations to their supervisor so a resident may possibly receive mental health services as soon as possible.

Family members can be a very valuable resource from which to gain information as it relates to a resident's mood, habits, routine, and personality prior to being admitted to the nursing home, and can also share any relevant psychiatric history to include psychiatric hospitalizations, however, this information must be solicited by nursing home staff for the information to be useful. Some residents and family members are very quick to volunteer this information, however, a great number of residents and family members are not sure what and how much information to share with the staff in a nursing home.

In most nursing homes, the social worker is generally the liaison between residents and family members who wish to discuss concerns related to residents' emotional and/or behavioral deficits. After listening too and validating information shared by residents and family members the social worker should then make referrals to the most appropriate health care providers to assist a resident and their family with resolving emotional and/or behavioral deficits. Remember, a resident who is cognitively intact and deemed able to make their own health care decisions and health care surrogates, proxies, guardians, must sign consent forms for a referral for mental health services.

While a social worker may be able to identify, address, and suggest that a resident in a nursing home seek appropriate mental health services, their efforts are sometimes thwarted by a resident's or health care surrogate's refusal of a referral to mental health services because they feel that a referral for mental health services would be admitting that a resident may be psychiatrically unstable.

Experiencing and admitting to emotional deficits can be a tough "pill" to swallow, especially for the sometimes macho male gender. Have you ever heard a geriatric individual say "I have lived a long life and I have never encountered a problem I couldn't solve myself"? This can be attributed to a defense mechanism know as denial that can often interfere with a resident receiving the appropriate care and treatment they require to alleviate their emotional and/or behavioral symptoms. Assisting a resident and/or family member work through denial can be most challenging for mental health professionals.

Clinical depression can have quite a devastating effect for a resident as it relates to emotional and/or physical deterioration. Decreased food/fluid intake related to symptoms to depression can lead to dehydration, electrolyte imbalances, gastric disorders, mental confusion, physical exhaustion, and in some cases, even death.

A resident in a nursing home that has capacity to make their own health care decisions has the right to refuse medical care. This often frustrates staff in nursing homes because they may feel they are not doing enough to help residents they are assigned too. Regardless of staff frustration, residents in nursing homes have a right to refuse care.

When a resident exercises their right to refuse care, they may be reassessed by their treating physician or ARNP to assess whether they can fully appreciate the medical, cognitive, and/or emotional consequences of their decision to refuse care. Lacking capacity to make ones own health care decisions is generally associated with being diagnosed with some form of dementia, however, I have seen a physician sign a "Lacks Capacity" form on a resident because the physician felt the resident could not fully appreciate the consequences of refusing medical and/or psychiatric care because the resident was severely depressed.

Remember, as we discussed in the chapter referring to Capacity, lacking capacity to make ones' own health care decisions can be a temporary situation. If a resident lacks capacity related to a psychiatric condition, once the resident is psychiatrically stabilized, the resident's treating physician should reassess the resident to readdress capacity to make their own health care decisions. Should a resident's assigned physician now feel the resident has capacity to make reasonable health care decisions ensure this information is recorded in the residents' medical record.

When a resident starts to lose weight, all medical causes should be ruled out as the cause of the weight loss. Weight loss in nursing homes can be indicative of underlying medical and/or psychiatric conditions. Once all medical causes are ruled out, one must consider psychiatric symptoms such as depression and/or anxiety that may be inducing weight loss. Unfortunately what occurs at times is weight loss is simply explained by someone in the nursing home stating "as people get older, they don't eat as much as they used too". As a resident or family member and you hear this reply, don't necessarily buy it.

Residents in nursing homes must have their weight recorded, usually on a monthly basis, unless there is cause to have a resident weighed more often. As a resident or family member of a resident, request to review the weight log for the previous three months so can also track a resident's body weight.

Anxiety is another psychiatric condition that can be debilitating for a resident in a nursing home. A resident experiencing symptoms of anxiety often have difficulty concentrating, have a disorganized and rambling thought process, have an inability to sit still resulting in episodes of restlessness and pacing, insomnia, short term memory impairment, fear of failing, rapid speech, and fatigue. They may lose the ability to make reasonable and realistic healthcare decisions and without treatment may not be able to return to their previous level of functioning.

Psychosis, whether it be a brief psychotic episode or related to a resident's diagnosis of dementia, can be extremely difficult to treat and stabilize in a nursing home setting. Some symptoms of psychotic behavior may include visual and/or auditory hallucinations, paranoia, delusional thought content (believing in something contrary to fact), aggression, and combative behavior directed at staff and/or other residents in the nursing home. Sometimes staff members in nursing homes become angry or frustrated when a resident becomes aggressive/violent, however, while most people fear aggression/violence, we must remember that a resident diagnosed with dementia generally cannot fully appreciate or comprehend the nature or consequences of their behavior.

Unfortunately, the most appropriate treatment for psychotic residents in nursing homes is the prescribing of psychotropic medications. I say unfortunate because psychotropic medications often have some serious side effects. Due to paranoia, a psychotic resident may refuse all their prescribed medications, firmly believing that the nurse that is administrating the medications is trying to poison them, and quite often, no amount of encouragement or coaxing will get a psychotic resident to take their prescribed medications. By refusing all prescribed medications, not just psychotropic medications, a psychotic resident is also compromising their medical status. The longer a psychotic resident refuses their medications, the longer the psychotic symptoms and behavioral deficits will persist.

Residents, health care surrogates/proxies and guardians often lack knowledge of medications, especially psychotropic medications. They are often unaware of the various side effects that accompany just about all medications. Before signing any forms that authorize the administration of medication, especially psychotropic medications, be sure to meet with the prescribing medical professional and request an explanation of the need for the medication, the desired therapeutic benefits, and the range of potential side effects of the various medications.

Psychotropic medications can be quite costly, therefore, if psychotropic medication is recommended and you have financial restraints, meet with the prescribing medical professional and assess whether another medication can be ordered that is less costly and/or contact a pharmacy to inquire as to the cost of a particular medication. For any individual that is prescribed medications, it would be in their best interest to purchase a Physician's Desk Reference Manual also known as a PDR) that contains information related to most medications because once you leave a meeting related to discussing medications, you can bet that you are more than likely to forget more than half of the information that was discussed related to medications. If you do not want to purchase a PDR, you can also request written information from your physician related to side effects of all medications that you are prescribed.

As a health care surrogate, you may receive a call from the physician, ARNP, social worker or nurse manager requesting an oral consent for a referral to mental health services. Should this occur, request a meeting with the resident's physician and any mental health professionals that may be available to inquire as to why a resident is in need of mental health care. Prior to the meeting, write down all questions you may have regarding mental health services and psychiatric medications you may have because without this list you will certainly leave the meeting with unanswered questions/concerns.

There are physicians that may feel somewhat uncomfortable prescribing psychotropic medications because psychiatry may not be their medical specialty, therefore, it would be in your best interest to become established as a patient of a psychiatrist of your choosing to prescribe and monitor your psychotropic medications. A psychiatrist may very well minimize or eliminate psychiatric symptoms in a shorter period of time than a general practitioner.

Family members are often overprotective of their loved ones, and given the moral, ethical and familial obligations they may feel toward family members, they are often in denial as to the capability of their loved one possibly injuring other residents or staff in a nursing home generally related to their diagnosis of dementia. Family members often lack education as it relates to behavioral disturbances residents with dementia often exhibit and lack insight into the fact that their loved one's behavior may become very unpredictable.

Ensuring the safety of all residents in a nursing home is no easy feat and is in no way guaranteed. The most that any nursing home can achieve is to ensure they have policies and procedures in place to minimize resident to resident abuse or residents' abuse of staff.

I have encountered several health care surrogates/proxies who authorized the use of physical and/or chemical restraints in the event their loved one had the potential to hurt others or who have already demonstrated aggressive/violent behavior toward others, however, state and federal guidelines prohibit nursing homes from using physical and/or chemical restraints to "control" a resident's mood and/or behavior deficits. Psychotropic medications can be considered a chemical restraint if not administered appropriately.

In summary, as a health care surrogate/proxy, or legal guardian, it would be of benefit to you to seek opportunities to become educated about the various needs, behaviors, and unpredictability of residents that are diagnosed with dementia and/or experiencing psychotic symptoms. If you are not sure where to seek educational information, be sure to request a meeting with the social worker who should be able to assist you with identifying referral sources to increase your awareness related to dementia and psychosis.

Alcohol and prescription drug use/abuse can certainly induce numerous problems for residents in nursing homes, as well as, the staff. When a resident resided at home, they may have enjoyed alcoholic beverages at times and now that they are in a nursing home, they find themselves missing their beverage of choice. If you are in this situation, do not panic. Schedule a meeting with your assigned physician and assess whether they would be willing to write an order that would permit you, as a resident, to have a couple of alcoholic beverages of your choice daily. Of course, this will depend on your medical status and what medications you may be prescribed. As a resident in a nursing home and you leave the facility to have dinner with your family, be careful if you drink any alcoholic beverages and, if you do, do not over imbibe. You certainly do not want to return to the nursing home inebriated.

When a resident was at home, they may have been prescribed a certain medication that they became accustomed to taking such as painkillers, sleeping pills, and over-the counter and now they find themselves in a nursing home, and for some reason, their physician will not prescribe the medication for them. Physicians have certain medications they have faith in and some they do not. As a resident, if you find yourself in this position, please do not encourage family members or visitors to bring you medications from outside of the facility. The medication they bring you may react adversely to the other medications you may be prescribed and you do not want to take a medication that your assigned physician is not aware of.

21

OMBUDSMAN'S COUNCIL

The Long Term Care Ombudsman Council is a group of folks whose goal is to improve/ensure the quality of life for residents in nursing homes including assisted living facilities. The long term care ombudsman is authorized to investigate complaints made by residents, family members, and health care surrogates and may assist a nursing home with an unruly resident they may wish to discharge from their facility.

An important role of the Ombudsman is to act as a mediator between residents, families, and employees of nursing homes when unsatisfactory events occur. A complaint to the ombudsman's council may be made in person, in writing, or by telephone and the complainant may remain anonymous if they so desire. It is better if the ombudsman knows who you are and how to contact you should they require additional information from you.

It is important to know that all information given to an Ombudsman is confidential unless a resident or complainant authorizes disclosure of the information. If you must be admitted to a nursing home, be sure to request a copy of the literature the nursing home has related to the services offered by the Long Term Ombudsman's Council. The Ombudsman is a very important resource as it relates to the quality of care residents receive in nursing homes.

22

PSYCHIATRIC HOSPITALIZATION

There are times when a resident's behavior cannot be managed and/or stabilized in a nursing home setting especially if a resident begins to physically abuse other residents in the nursing home, as well as, staff.

There are generally two avenues for a resident in a nursing home to be admitted to an inpatient psychiatric facility. One is on a voluntary basis, and the other an involuntary basis. Laws governing voluntary versus involuntary admission to a psychiatric hospital may vary from state to state.

A resident in a nursing home that has capacity to make their own health care decisions, has not been diagnosed with a form of dementia, and has insight into their need for inpatient psychiatric care may voluntarily admit themselves to an inpatient psychiatric facility. If a resident in a nursing home lacks capacity to make reasonable health care decisions and/ or has been diagnosed with dementia, generally cannot be admitted to an inpatient psychiatric facility on a voluntary basis and, if required, will have to be admitted to a psychiatric facility on an involuntary basis.

In the state of Florida for instance, an appointed health care surrogate or proxy cannot authorize admission for a resident to a psychiatric facility on a voluntary basis, however, once a resident is involuntarily admitted to an inpatient psychiatric facility, the health care surrogate retains the right to make health care decisions for the resident. Be sure to research the laws in your state related to involuntary psychiatric hospitalization for a resident diagnosed with dementia and what your rights are as a resident's appointed health care surrogate.

In most states, a law enforcement officer, physician, and certain licensed mental health professionals may initiate involuntary hospitalization for a resident in a nursing home if the resident is deemed a possible danger to themselves or others. This can be tricky at times because the individual who initiates a petition for involuntary psychiatric hospitalization of a nursing home resident must have witnessed the resident exhibiting behaviors that may be considered a danger to themselves or others and cannot initiate an involuntary petition on hearsay or second hand information. This does not always occur. There also must be adequate clinical documentation to substantiate the need for involuntary psychiatric hospitalization. Nursing homes have had difficulty ensuring that staff document all episodes of aggressive behavior exhibited by a resident in their care and as the old saying goes, "if it is not documented, it didn't occur".

While being considered a danger to yourself and/or others related to aggressive behavior is the criteria that must be met before a petition for involuntary psychiatric hospitalization is initiated, another scenario that meets the criteria for involuntary psychiatric hospitalization is self-neglect.

One may ask "how can a resident suffer from self-neglect when they reside in a nursing home and have entrusted their care needs to health care professionals"? Remember, a resident in a nursing home that has capacity to make their own health care decisions has the right, under law, to refuse medical care. At times, this can induce quite a dilemma for health care providers because while they must be cognizant of resident's rights as it relates to refusing medical care, they must also make medical judgments as to whether a resident's refusal of care constitutes self-neglect.

As a health care provider in a nursing home, when a resident refuses medical care, it is very important that you do your best to try and assess the reason/reasons why a resident is refusing medical care. A resident may refuse care simply because they are having a bad day, may have a urinary tract infection that may induce confusion in the elderly population, or may be depressed. When a resident begins refusing medical care in a nursing home, the resident's treating physician should reassess a resident's capacity to make reasonable and realistic health care decisions. Should the physician feel that the resident continues to have capacity to make their own health care decisions and a resident continues to refuse medical care that may compromise their medical status, the physician may initiate a Baker Act and a resident can then be admitted to an inpatient psychiatric facility on an involuntary basis secondary to self-neglect. It is very important that staff document all episodes of refusing care in a resident's clinical record.

As a resident in a nursing home with capacity to make your own health care decisions or the health care surrogate/ proxy or guardian of a resident that lacks capacity to make their own health care decisions, it is very important that you meet with the physician, social worker, or a mental health professional if the nursing home employs one to review all documentation of aggressive behavior and/or episodes of refusing care.

This can be tricky because while cognitively intact residents in a nursing home have the right to refuse care, if a resident's treating physician or the Administrator feels that a resident's needs cannot be met in their nursing home because of aggressive behavior, refusal of care, or self-neglect that puts the resident or others in possible danger, the administrator may issue the resident or their health care surrogate a thirty day notice of transfer/discharge from the nursing home of which a copy is forwarded to the Ombudsman's office. Given this information, do not be too quick to refuse care while exercising your right to do so.

With HIPAA guidelines in place as it relates to confidentiality of information, a nursing home must really be on their toes as to what information they are permitted to share and to whom. If issued a thirty day notice of transfer or discharge, when another nursing home is located and they "catch wind" that a resident was issued a thirty day notice of transfer/discharge from another nursing home because they could not meet their medical and/or psychiatric care needs, they may be unwilling to admit a resident to their nursing home unless the census in the nursing home is low and they are willing to "take a chance" on a resident with a history of unacceptable behavior.

If a resident in a nursing home is issued a thirty day notice of transfer/discharge from a nursing home, be sure to meet with the social worker for assistance in locating another nursing home. If as a resident with capacity or a health care surrogate, you disagree with the nursing home for, whatever reason, with being issued a thirty day notice of transfer/discharge from a nursing home, you have the right to request a hearing with the Ombudsman to ensure that your rights are being protected and to ensure that the nursing home simply does not want you as a resident in their nursing home.

While most nursing homes strive to honor the wishes of residents and family members, medical professionals who are providing the care a resident requires and in whom a resident has entrusted their care must always remain cognizant of who is directing resident care, the medical professionals, the resident, their family, or a health care surrogate.

23

PRESSURE ULCERS
(Bed Sores)

Also known as decubitus ulcers, it is essentially a breakdown in a resident's skin integrity generally caused by continuous pressure on the skin where the skin comes in contact with surfaces such as seats and backs of wheelchairs and the mattress on the bed. Common areas where skin breakdown may occur include the buttocks, coccyx, elbows, and heels. Skin breakdown can also result from improper peri-care (cleaning of the genital area) after a resident has a bowel movement or experiences an episode of bowel and/or bladder incontinence.

There are essentially four stages of pressure ulcers: **Stage 1**—a persistent area of skin redness without a break in the skin that does not disappear when pressure is relieved. **Stage 2**—a partial thickness loss of skin that presents clinically as an abrasion, blister, or shallow crater. **Stage 3**—when a full thickness of skin is lost, exposing subcutaneous tissues and presents as a deep crater with or without undermining adjacent tissue. **Stage 4**—A full thickness of skin and subcutaneous tissue is lost, exposing muscle or bone.

Stage three and four pressure ulcers can be quite poten-tially dangerous related to infection and may require a long time to heal and may also require surgery and you can only hope that a resident with a stage three or four pressure ulcer that requires surgery is a surgical candidate related to other medical complications. Most nursing homes either have an in-house wound care nurse or they contract with would care professionals to treat pressure ulcers and to monitor the heal-ing process.

Residents in nursing homes that, for whatever reason, spend most of their time in bed are encouraged to turn themselves every two to three hours to distribute the pressure that is applied to their skin when spending to much time in bed. If a resident is unable to turn themselves every two hours because of medical and/or cognitive deficits, it is the responsibility of the nursing staff to ensure that a resident is turned at least every two to three hours, however, this does not always occur and as a result, a resident may be at risk for developing skin breakdown and a subsequent pressure ulcer.

Nursing homes start to become quite concerned when res-idents develop pressure ulcers "in-house" as pressure ulcers are closely monitored by state nursing home surveyors and could possibly indicate substandard care.

If pressure ulcers occur to often in a nursing home, state surveyors may investigate and if they feel that a nursing home is providing substandard care, they may issue a moratorium on new admissions until such a time when they have concluded that the problem has been resolved. At the extreme, the state can order a nursing home to close their doors and will have their nursing home license suspended or revoked. When this occurs, locating nursing homes to relocate residents too can be quite a difficult task. Large fines may also be imposed on a nursing home that has had their license suspended or revoked.

As a resident or family member of a resident in a nursing home that develops a pressure ulcer in-house, meet with the Director of Nursing to ensure that an investigation as to how and why a pressure ulcer developed is underway. If you are given what you consider "lame" reasons/excuses as to how a pressure ulcer developed, remember, you always have the right to contact your Ombudsman's office and request their intervention.

Examining a resident's skin PRIOR to being admitted to a nursing home is very important so you and the nursing home staff can be assured that a resident was not admitted to the nursing home with a pressure ulcer. Upon admission to a nursing home, a resident has a skin assessment conducted by the nursing staff. After the skin assessment is completed, meet with the nurse to assess whether you missed anything when you conducted your own skin assessment.

As a resident or family member, examine your/their skin on a very regular basis to observe for signs/symptoms associated with pressure ulcers. Should you discover areas of skin that may be suspect for skin breakdown, meet with the Nurse Manager or the Director of Nursing to ensure that treatment begins promptly.

24

RESIDENT ABUSE

The abuse of residents in nursing homes is inappropriate, unacceptable, and illegal and is not tolerated by reputable nursing homes. Emotional abuse is when one verbally belittles a resident, ignores a resident's request, and presents as unsympathetic to a resident's plight. Physical abuse is handling residents in a rough manner resulting in bruising and/or fractures or slapping/pushing a resident. It can also induce fear in a resident. Sexual abuse is touching a resident in a manner that is considered inappropriate, fondling a resident, or having sexual relations with a resident. Neglect is not responding to residents' requests, not meeting residents' physical and/or emotional needs such as allowing a resident to lay in soiled sheets or incontinence briefs for extended periods of time, and not assisting a resident with feeding when they are unable to feed themselves. The above are only some examples of neglect. Other situations may arise that constitutes neglect. Exploitation is making gain out of or at the expense of another person whether it may be money, possessions, or services. Requesting and/or convincing a resident to include you in their Last Will and Testament is a classic example of exploitation.

As a visitor or family member of a resident in a nursing home and you notice a bruise on a resident, please do not overreact, jump to conclusions, and/or become convinced that the resident was "definitely" physically abused. I am not suggesting that you take it lightly either. Should you notice a bruise on your friend or family member in a nursing home, request a meeting with the resident's assigned nurse, as well as, the nurse manager on duty to assess the possible origin of the bruise and to assess whether they even knew that the resident had a bruise, skin tear, etc.

After consulting with the nurse and nurse manager about possible causes for the bruise, process the information they shared and, if it is your impression that they may have presented as vague while discussing possible causes for a bruise or skin tear, and/or have difficulty accepting their explanations, request a meeting with the Director of Nursing to further discuss this issue.

When you visit your friend or family member in a nursing home and it is your impression that almost every time you visit, they have fresh bruises or skin tears, this should send up a "red flag" that the resident may be subjected to abuse by the staff and/or another resident.

At this point, I would suggest meeting with the nurse manager and the Director of Nursing and the Administrator of the nursing home to further discuss and investigate why a resident is being bruised or sustains skin tears on a very frequent basis. Remember, if not content with their position and/or explanations they provide, you have the right to contact the Ombudsman's office.

Visitors and family members must realize that residents in nursing homes often sustain bruising and/or other injuries due to no fault on the staff's part. As we grow older, our skin may become quite thin and tear easily. At times, residents in nursing home scratch and pick at their skin that may result in skin tears. Residents often mishandle their walkers/wheelchairs and collide with furniture, walls, other wheelchairs, and ambulatory residents, resulting in injury. A visually impaired resident may constantly run/bump into things. A major cause of serious injuries to residents is the failure of cognitively impaired residents to use their walker and wheelchairs.

Residents in nursing homes often hurt themselves while in bed with the side rails in the up position to prevent them from falling/rolling out of bed. They often hit the side rails with their hands, arms, and legs that result in bruising or skin tears. Some resident have fractured their arms by getting their arm tangled up in a bed rail. I have had family members instruct the staff to leave the side rails down when a resident is in bed so they do not hurt themselves because of the side rails however should a resident's treating physician feel that a resident lacks knowledge of bed boundaries and may sustain serious injury such as fractures and head trauma should they fall out of bed, the side rails will be in the up position while the resident is in bed. If a resident lacks knowledge of bed boundaries and falls out of bed sustaining injury, this could represent neglect on the staff's part for failure to ensure that the side rails were in the raised position when the resident was in the bed.

If a resident falls while using the toilet, and it is common knowledge that the resident requires assistance with toileting, as established by the nursing staff and the resident's care plan team, it is more than likely the resident was left on the toilet without staff supervision or the resident attempted to toilet themselves without the assistance they require. Not only does a care plan team determine that a resident requires assistance with toileting, they also determine whether it takes one or two certified nursing assistants to help a resident with toileting. Given this scenario, it may be difficult for family members to accept and/or understand why a resident fell in the bathroom while being toileted.

As a family member, should you suspect ongoing abuse of residents in a nursing home, you can contact the Ombudsman's office and/or you can relocate your family member to another nursing home. Every nursing home must post the phone number of the Abuse Registry in a common area that permits individuals to report actual or suspected abuse of residents in nursing homes.

Most nursing homes are diligent as it relates to ensuring adequate background screening for new staff and most staff members employed in nursing homes are honest, hard working individuals who would never entertain the idea of abusing, neglecting, or exploiting a resident entrusted in their care. As a staff member in a nursing home, should you observe another staff member abusing, neglecting, or exploiting a resident, you are bound by law to report such abuse.

25

RESIDENT/FAMILY COUNCIL MEETING

State regulations require nursing homes to conduct monthly resident council meetings that afford residents in nursing homes a forum to share their thoughts, feelings, etc. related to the services residents receive in a nursing home. This is also an opportunity for resident to suggest improvements as it relates to the delivery of services in the nursing home. The activity department in a nursing home generally hosts the resident council meeting.

It would be in their best interests for nursing homes to heed residents suggestions as it relates to improving the delivery of service in the nursing home because a member of the yearly survey team will be sure to attend a resident council meeting and/or will poll residents individually to assess whether the nursing home is open/receptive to considering suggestions for improving the services provided by the nursing home. Believe me when I say residents in nursing homes are not very shy when it comes to sharing their thoughts and feelings with state surveyors. As a resident in a nursing home, it at all possible, it would certainly be to your advantage to attend the monthly resident council meetings.

Nursing homes generally also conduct monthly or quarterly family council meetings. Ideally, the meeting should be of an educational nature as it relates to issues considered important to the geriatric population. At times, family council meetings get "off track" and often become a forum for repetitive complaints about issues related to services provided by the nursing home. As a family member attending a family council meeting, assist the nursing home in maintaining the purpose/goal of the meeting, which should be an educational experience. If a family member has concerns about care issues, take your concerns directly to the Nurse Manager, the Assistant Director of Nursing, the Director of Nursing, and/or the Administrator of the nursing home.

26

RESIDENT RELOCATION

As a former social worker in a nursing home, relocating residents to other rooms, units, etc. within the facility was one of my most challenging experiences as it relates to seeking authorization from a resident, health care surrogate/proxy or legal guardian to relocate a resident to another room or unit within the nursing home.

Admissions representatives or marketing representatives of nursing homes do not always obtain as much information about a perspective admission prior to agreeing to admit a resident to their nursing home. Unfortunately, this may occur because the nursing home is to quick to "fill a bed" due to budgeting issues, and as a result, sometimes numerous problems occur and new admissions find themselves dealing with the relocation process shortly after admission.

It would certainly be in the best interest of a nursing home to take the time to conduct an adequate, acceptable assessment on a perspective new admission because they are well aware that once a resident is in their nursing home, it can be quite difficult to relocate or discharge a "problem" resident from the nursing home, not to mention the emotional impact the relocation or discharge process may have on a resident and their family. Newly admitted residents that are diagnosed with dementia and/or psychosis or have an extensive psychiatric history, will certainly experience great difficulty adjusting to their new environment.

If a resident with capacity to make their own health care decisions requests relocation to another room for whatever reason, this is usually relatively easy to accomplish. On many occasions, health care surrogates are very reluctant to agree to relocation for their resident because they feel that relocating the resident to another room or unit may only further confuse the resident. Sometimes, this is very true, however, as a resident, a health care surrogate/proxy or legal guardian of a resident in a nursing home, be sure to meet with the staff at the nursing home who are seeking your authorization for relocation and do your best to ensure that the nursing home is not requesting the relocation simply for their convenience. Should this occur, refuse the nursing home's request to relocate to another room or unit within the facility. If the nursing home puts to much pressure on you to authorize the relocation of a resident, remember, you always have the right to contact the Ombudsman's office for assistance.

Sometimes residents, family members, health care surrogates/proxies and legal guardians are very rigid individuals and no matter what length one goes to please them, they will never be satisfied. If an Administrator feels that they must relocate a resident to another room or unit of the nursing home to ensure the safety of a resident and all residents in their nursing home, you can bet that the "problem" resident will more than likely be relocated to another room or unit without the consent of the resident, family member, health care surrogate/proxy or legal guardian. **REMEMBER**, the Ombudsman's Council can also assist nursing homes with resolving difficult issues with residents and family members.

In some instances, resident relocation within a nursing home is necessary and appropriate. If you are occupying a Medicare bed in a nursing home and are decertified from Medicare but must remain in the nursing home for whatever reason, you will be required to relocate to a bed that is not Medicare certified so the nursing home can be assured there will be an available Medicare bed for a new admission to the Medicare unit, also referred to as the acute care unit.

Should a resident in a nursing home become an elopement risk, they may be required to relocate to another area of the nursing home where the resident can be supervised more closely and cannot leave their unit or the nursing home without being accompanied by staff, family members, or visitors. Before relocating a resident who is considered an elopement risk, other measures should be attempted first such as requiring the resident to wear some form of monitoring device on their person that sounds an alarm to alert staff should the resident attempt to leave their unit or nursing home unaccompanied or the resident hires a private duty aide who will accompany the resident off the unit or outside the nursing home.

Resident safety should be the number one priority of all nursing homes. Should your loved one in a nursing home become an elopement risk, meet with the nurse manager or the social worker and be sure they obtain a monitoring device specifically designed and indicated for residents in nursing homes that pose an elopement risk.

A very tricky area for a social worker in a nursing home is when a married couple reside in a nursing home, however, they do not share a room together because one or both, or a health care surrogate, have requested they not share a room together. Most people would assume that a married couple in a nursing home would share a room together after all they may have been married for many years. Another assumption most people would make is that because a couple have been married for many years, they must have had a wonderful marriage. This is not always the case.

One of the couple may have moderate to severe cognitive impairment and may not recognize their spouse any longer while the other may be cognitively intact and to share a room together may cause numerous problems for the cognitively intact partner.

A resident may have great difficulty sharing their reasons as to why they do not want to share a room with their spouse and should they share their reasons with you as a health care provider, you must keep this information confidential. This information could be emotionally devastating to their spouse if released. Withholding confidential information from family members, when they request information, may cause them quite a bit of frustration, however, they must realize that a resident has a right to confidentiality for their own reasons.

Should this occur, the most a health care provider can do is to share with a resident that their family members are having quite a bit of difficulty understanding and/or accepting they may not want to share a room with their spouse and then it is up to the resident to decide what information they want to remain confidential and what information can be shared with others.

A spouse may not know why they are not sharing a room with their spouse because no one has shared this information with them for whatever reason. When a resident inquires of you as a health care professional as to why they are not sharing a room with their spouse, and you have been requested by the resident who does not want to reside with their spouse to keep their reasons confidential, at times, this puts nursing home staff in a very difficult position. While staff must always be as honest as possible with residents in nursing homes, one must become somewhat creative as how to respond to the resident's inquiry as to why they are not sharing a room with their spouse. This would be an appropriate time to attempt to enlist the family's assistance and support in this matter. Residents in nursing homes are generally more receptive to suggestions made by their family than the staff of a nursing home. Family members may not be bound by confidentially laws that apply to staff in nursing homes, however, should they release information that a resident requested be held confidential, they may run the risk of losing a resident's trust.

Should a resident with capacity or the health care surrogate/proxy or legal guardian of a resident who lacks capacity to make their own health care decision should you feel that it would not be in the best interest of a married couple to share a room together in a nursing home, the facility should ensure that this information is very well documented in the medical records of the married couple because when the nursing home has their annual survey, the survey team is certainly going to expect an acceptable response as to why a married couple in the nursing home are not sharing a room together.

If the appropriate information is not well documented as to why a married couple are not sharing a room together this can create a very uncomfortable situation for a nursing home that may result in a violation of resident's rights and a fine may be imposed on the nursing home. A nursing home should be cited by state surveyors if their documentation is inadequate, however, if the documentation is adequate and accurate, the nursing home should come out of the potential conflict relatively unscathed.

27

RESIDENTS RIGHTS

All residents in nursing homes have certain rights that the staff and the nursing home are legally responsible to acknowledge and to ensure that these rights are honored and protected.

Below are the rights that residents enjoy and are entitled too while residing in a nursing home:

1. You have the right to be fully informed of your total health status, including your current medical status;

2. You have the right to be fully informed in advance of your medical care and treatment, any changes in such care and treatment;

3. You have the right to have your family and physician promptly notified of significant changes in your medical condition and/or status;

4. You have the right to be informed of services available to you, and the related charges for such services;

5. You have the right to be informed on how to apply for and use Medicare and Medicaid benefits;

6. You have the right to be informed on how to receive a refund from previous payments covered by Medicare;

7. You have the right to be informed of the name, specialty, and way of contacting the physician responsible for your medical care;

8. You have the right to choose a personal attending physician;

9. You have the right to refuse your nursing care and medical treatment, and to refuse to participate in any experimental research;

10. You have the right to self-administer your drugs and medications if the care plan team determines it is safe;

11. You have the right to personal privacy;

12. You have the right to privacy in receiving and sending written communication;

13. You have the right to retain and use personal possessions;

14. You have the right to have regular access to the private use of a telephone;

15. You have the right to exercise your rights as a resident of the facility;

16. You have the right to receive visitors at any time;

17. You have the right to interact with members of the community;

18. You have the right to choose activities, schedules, and care consistent with your interests, assessment, and plan of care;

19. You have the right to receive services with reasonable accommodation of individual needs and preferences;

20. You have a right to be notified of a change in your room assignment or roommate;

21. You have a right to share a room with your spouse should both of you be residents in the facility;

22. You have the right to be free from verbal, physical, sexual, and mental abuse, or exploitation, corporal punishment, and involuntary seclusion;

23. You have the right to be free from interference, coercion, discrimination or reprisal from the facility in exercising your rights;

24. You have the right to contact and receive information from agencies acting as resident advocates;

25. You have the right to be free from physical and chemical restraints;

26. You have the right to be fully informed of your rights;

27. You have the right to be fully informed, orally and in writing, of your responsibilities to the facility;

28. You have the right to receive written copies of any change(s) in rules and regulations that may affect your rights, obligations, or responsibilities to the facility;

29. You have the right to be informed of the facility's bed-hold policy;

30. You have the right to receive a 30-day notice before transferred or discharged from the facility;

31. You have the right to manage your own financial affairs;

32. You have the right to file a grievance, and/or complaint with the facility, state survey and certification agency,

ombudsman, or other advocates concerning abuse, neglect, or misappropriation of your personal property.

33. You have the right to inspect and purchase photocopies of your records;

34. You have the right to confidentiality of your personal and clinical records;

35. You have the right to examine the most recent survey report and the facility's plan of correction;

36. You have the right to refuse to perform or not perform services for the facility;

37. You have the right to organize and participate in resident groups in the facility;

38. You have the right to participate in social, religious, and community activities;

39. You have the right to make choices about aspects of your life in the facility.

These are your rights as a resident in a nursing home. Please take the time to learn your rights and do not hesitate to exercise your rights in a nursing home because do not assume that the nursing home staff will ensure that your resident rights are enforced and protected.

If at any time, you believe that you have been subjected to abuse, neglect, or exploitation, while a resident in a nursing home, and/or you feel that your resident rights have not been honored, contact the Abuse Hotline number that must be posted in a very visible location in every nursing home, as well as, contacting your local Ombudsman and request their intervention.

28

ROOMMATES

If your finances are such that you cannot afford a private room in a nursing home, you will have to share a semi-private room with another resident. If the nursing home is diligent related to roommate compatibility, it can certainly minimize problems between roommates and hopefully will provide comfort and reassurance to their families.

In a semi-private room, you will now find yourself sharing a room with a total stranger and you are going to initially experience some problems until you have had sufficient time to learn more about your roommates' personality, habits, etc. For a short-term resident, this is a short-term issue however, for some permanent residents in nursing homes they will always now have a roommate. This will certainly have a major life changing effect on some residents.

Compatibility factors generally include a resident's personality, habits, toileting needs, dietary issues, sleeping patterns, and medical and cognitive status. It would not be wise to place two residents together that require extensive toileting assistance. The bathroom would be tied up for quite a long time. It is not wise to place residents together when one enjoys staying up late watching television while the other enjoys going to sleep early in the evening. You may consider this a common sense approach, however, residents in nursing homes get placed together that exhibit the habits mentioned above.

If a resident is cognitively intact and is placed with a resident with moderate to severe cognitive impairment, problems will certainly arise. You may return to your room and observe your roommate rummaging through your possessions or laying/sleeping in your bed. You may also notice some of your clothes missing, as well as, your glasses, dentures, or hearing aids. While this may upset you, remember that a cognitively impaired resident may not be aware that they are exhibiting inappropriate behavior. The cognitively intact resident will more than likely not receive the social interaction and conversational stimulation they enjoy and require when sharing a room with a cognitively impaired resident.

Sometimes, two friends in a nursing home may request to be placed together in the same room however, at times they engage in disagreements and request to be separated. While efforts may be made to satisfy such a request, a resident may have to wait until a bed is available with a more compatible roommate and this may take a while. Just because two residents may consider themselves friends does not ensure that they will be compatible roommates.

We must also remember that roommates are going to change from time to time. As a resident on the Medicare unit your roommate may be discharged to home soon and you will be getting a new roommate rather quickly because in some nursing homes there may be a very strong demand for Medicare beds. Your present roommate may pass away or you may be relocated to another room on the Medicare unit to accommodate a resident's need for isolation or to allow a married couple to be able to share a room.

Residents and family members often inquire of staff as to their roommates medical and/or cognitive status, habits, behaviors, etc., however, as a resident or family member, remember that nursing home staff are mandated by law to ensure the confidentiality of information related to the residents in their facility and more than likely may not share this information with you. This may bother you as a resident or family member but ensuring confidentiality of a resident's medical and personal information is paramount in the health care field.

Many staff members have been terminated due to breaching confidentiality guidelines. As a resident or family member, you will generally obtain information when you interact with your roommate, their family members, and visitors.

Should you as a resident or health care surrogate of a resident feel that there are moderate to severe compatibility issues between roommates, schedule to meet with the nurse manager and the social worker to discuss a possible relocation to another room and hopefully a more compatible roommate.

29

SEXUAL NEEDS AND EXPRESSION

For decades, a large part of the geriatric population were under the impression that when men started to develop prostate problems and women experienced menopause, nature dictated that sexual drives and expression no longer existed.

Many of today's geriatric population were schooled in such a fashion that to even discuss sexual thoughts and feelings were considered taboo. Physical contact between the sexes, whether it be holding hands or hugging a member of the opposite sex who is not a family member, was often viewed as a "public spectacle". Society has come a long way since then as it relates to acceptance of public displays of affection. Regardless of the attitudes about sexual or physical expression decades ago or in the present, most people have a basic need to touch, as well as, to be touched by others, including members of the opposite sex. For some elderly folks, their need to touch others and be touched is often suppressed because of depression and/or anxiety.

Have you ever heard adult children tell their parents they are acting like "kids again" because they may be more open, verbally and physically, when sharing their feelings for each other?

As a child, did you have a particular aunt or grandmother that you did not like to visit because every time you visited her, she would give you a big hug and plant a big, wet, kiss on your cheek or forehead that you wanted to immediately rub off? As you matured, you may have begun to recognize and understand that your aunt and grandmother were simply expressing their need to give and receive a hug from someone most dear to them. The part touch plays in offering encouragement and emotional support, as well as feelings of love and tenderness can be quite rewarding.

When a spouse dies, the surviving spouse may find themselves somewhat isolated from others and may now be without transportation, restricting contact with family and friends to obtain the physical contact and emotional support they desire and require. When denied physical contact with friends and family, the elderly often become shut-ins and feel helpless and hopeless. They may become somewhat confused and unsure as to how to rebuild their social structure.

Inappropriate touching or sexual behavior exhibited by residents in nursing homes that lack capacity and present with moderate to severe cognitive impairment is another issue. Let's not forget that cognitively impaired residents in nursing homes also require and enjoy human touch that makes them feel good and secure. We must also remember that cognitively impaired residents often do not realize they are exhibiting inappropriate sexual behavior. Cognitively impaired residents often do not understand the concept of "informed consent" and often attempt to engage in some form of sexual activity with residents who are not receptive to their advances and may become more confused, depressed and/or agitated when their sexual advances are rebuffed. Not being able to reason with a moderate to severely cognitively impaired resident certainly puts restrictions on treatment and intervention alternatives that may result in psychotropic medications and/or libido reducing medications being prescribed.

As a spouse visiting their spouse in a nursing home and you observe your spouse touching another resident in a way you consider inappropriate, although it may have quite an emotional impact on you, do not become enraged for your cognitively impaired spouse may not be aware that their behavior may be considered inappropriate because of some form of dementia. As a spouse, observing your spouse exhibiting inappropriate behavior with other residents in the nursing home may be emotionally devastating for you, however, becoming angry with your spouse, attempting to reason with your spouse, and requesting that they cease the inappropriate behavior may be of no benefit because their spouse's short term memory deficit prevents them from retaining new information that is shared with them.

Should you visit your spouse in a nursing home and they are exhibiting behavior that you consider inappropriate, inform the staff and permit them to calmly redirect your spouse to some form of more appropriate activity. You should also schedule time to meet with the resident's assigned physician to discuss possible treatment interventions to hopefully manage and/or eliminate inappropriate behavior exhibited by your spouse.

30

STAFF ROLES

As a resident, or the family member of a resident in a nursing home, it is very important to become acquainted with the staff and learn the responsibilities of each discipline so when a problem arises, you will know who to meet with to hopefully resolve your concerns. Outlined below are the various disciplines employed by nursing homes and a brief description of their responsibilities/duties.

ADMINISTRATOR: is ultimately responsible to ensure that the delivery of services within the nursing home meets or exceeds current state regulations. One of their primary responsibilities is to ensure that the nursing home provides the necessary services within the budget allotted for the nursing home.

The Administrator oversees department heads that are responsible for ensuring that the staff provides health care services in a competent, professional, and caring manner. The Administrator is the individual that residents, family members, health care surrogates, and staff should contact when they have issues to address and have "worked through" the chain of command with unsatisfactory results.

DIRECTOR OF NURSING (DON): supervises the Assistant Director of Nursing and nurse managers to ensure that the staff they supervise are providing necessary care to the residents in a kind, competent, and professional manner. The DON is responsible for the delivery of services in the nursing home as it relates to all nursing functions within the nursing home. The DON reports directly to the Administrator.

ASSISTANT DIRECTOR OF NURSING (ADON); reports directly to the DON and supervises the nurse managers to ensure they are performing their duties accurately and professionally and are properly supervising the staff they are assigned too. The ADON is generally responsible for the delivery of service as it relates to nursing services in the absence of the DON. The ADON reports directly to the DON.

NURSE MANAGER: is responsible for ensuring that the unit nurses and the certified nursing assistants they are assigned too perform their duties in a caring, competent, and professional manner. The nurse manager reports directly to the ADON or the DON if the nursing home does not have an ADON position.

UNIT NURSE: is responsible for ensuring the certified nursing assistants assigned to them are performing their duties in a competent, caring, professional manner and is responsible for ensuring that the medical needs of their assigned residents are met. The unit nurse reports directly to the nurse manager they are assigned too. The unit nurse may be either an LPN or an RN. Many nursing homes employ LPN's, as opposed to RN's, because they can save quite a bit of money as LPN's are not as financially compensated as RN's.

However, nursing homes are mandated by state regulations as to the number of RN's that must be present in the nursing home at any given time. Some nursing homes will meet the minimum standards required by law related to RN's being on duty so they can meet their budgetary goals however some nursing homes hold themselves to a higher standard and will exceed the minimum guidelines.

CERTIFIED NURSING ASSISTANT (CNA): provides most of the direct care services within a nursing home to include assisting residents with transferring them in and out of bed, in and out of a wheelchair, and on and off the toilet. They also assist residents with their dressing, toileting, hygiene and grooming needs, and bathing needs, as well as, setting up meal trays for residents who are able to feed themselves and feeding residents that are unable to feed themselves. They report directly to their assigned unit nurse.

CERTIFIED DIETARY MANAGER: they have a tremendous responsibility ensuring that all meals leave the kitchen hot, according to schedule, and to ensure that the proper menu selections are delivered to the proper residents and the proper meal carts are delivered to the proper units within the nursing home.

REGISTERED DIETICIAN: is responsible for ensuring that all residents in the nursing home are prescribed nutritious, therapeutic diets. They consult with the speech therapist to discuss a resident's ability to swallow that may result in dietary changes.

DIRECTOR OF ACTIVITIES: if a nursing is large enough, they may also have activity assistants. They are responsible to ensure that the social and activity needs of all residents in the nursing home are met on a daily basis.

PHYSICAL THERAPIST : works with residents in nursing homes that require rehabilitation as it relates to post operative joint replacements, stroke victims, and residents with gait (ambulating) disturbances .They also perform other valuable services in their quest to assist a resident with attaining and maintaining their prior level of functioning.

OCCUPATIONAL THERAPIST: works with residents in nursing homes to be as independent as possible with activities of daily living such as dressing, toileting, hygiene/ grooming, and bathing needs.

Should in-home physical and/or occupational therapy be indicated post discharge from a nursing home, an in-home evaluation is very important to assess the safety of the environment to where you are being discharged. The home health agency that will be responsible for providing your in-home therapy would more than likely be the agency that would assess the safety of your home environment to assess if durable medical equipment is required in the home such as grab bars in the shower, high toilet seat, shower chair, hospital bed, wheelchair, etc. and they would make the arrangements to have the durable medical equipment delivered and hopefully installed in your home. The social worker in a nursing home can also order durable medical equipment for your home in consultation with the home health agency. Throw rugs and furniture not placed strategically in a home can contribute to increased falls resulting in injury and may also restrict ambulation and mobility in the home.

SPEACH THERAPIST: works closely with residents to assist them in regaining speech deficits related to stroke symptoms and other medical disorders. They consult with the Registered Dietician to ensure that residents are prescribed diets and liquids they can tolerate.

PHYSICIAN/ARNP: nursing homes generally have an in-house physician or they contract with a local physician to provide medical services to the residents in their facility. Ideally, a nursing home should contract with a physician who has considerable geriatric experience because they will have to treat residents who present with age related medical and cognitive issues, as well as, mood and/or behavioral deficits. Some nursing homes employ an ARNP (Advanced Registered Nurse Practitioner) who may be able to spend more time in the nursing home caring for residents than a contract physician. An ARNP is authorized to prescribe medications and works very closely with the physician that is providing medical services to the nursing home, as well as, with the staff in the nursing home.

CHAPLAIN: some nursing may employ an in-house chaplain to ensure that the religious/spiritual needs of the residents and their family members are being met. If a nursing home does not have an in-house chaplain, they must make every effort to ensure that pastoral services are available to their residents, regardless of a resident's religious affiliation. As a resident, you have the right to have your own priest, pastor, or rabbi visit you in the nursing home to meet your religious or spiritual needs.

SOCIAL WORKER: works closely with residents, family members, and all departments in a nursing home to ensure that a resident is receiving the professional care they are entitled too. They are generally responsible for obtaining copies of residents Advanced Medical Directives to include their code status (DNR versus Full Code status), ensure that residents rights are enforced, assist residents with adjusting to nursing home placement, address resident relocation within the facility, assist residents with locating another nursing home should they be issued a thirty day notice of discharge from the facility, coordinate and arrange psychiatric services, and most importantly, are generally the liaison between the nursing home, family members, health care surrogates and health care agencies in the community.

As a resident, family member, or health care surrogate, when a problem with care in a nursing home occurs be sure that you are discussing your concerns with the appropriate staff members who can hopefully help you resolve your concerns. Remember that if the staff member you are meeting with is of no assistance in helping you resolve your concerns, go the next highest level in the "chain of command".

WORKSHEET

(USE PENCIL)

Staff Member:

Administrator: _____

DON:

_____

ADON: _____

**Nurse
Manager:** _____

**Unit
Nurse:** _____

Clinical Dietician: _____

Certified Dietary Manager: _____

Director of Activities: _____

Physical Therapist: _____

Occupational Therapist: _____

Speech Therapist: _____

Physician/Arnp: _____

Chaplain: _____

Social Worker: _____

31

STATE SURVEY

Oh boy, what a time this is for nursing homes. A nursing home generally does not know what day a state survey team will arrive for their annual survey however, they generally have about a three month window period when they can be assured that the survey team will arrive. It has been my experience that when a state survey team is in the local area, local nursing homes call other nursing homes to give them a "head's up" that the survey team is in the area.

Once this occurs, a nursing home will generally conduct meetings with the staff and share that the survey team could arrive any day and they should really "be on their toes" as it relates to the delivery of services they provide to their residents. When a state survey team arrives at a nursing home, they will generally post a notice in the lobby of the nursing home announcing their arrival and the estimated length of time it will require to conduct their inspection/survey. The survey usually takes about three to four days.

The survey team generally consists of RN's, a Social Worker, a Registered Dietician, and a building inspector.

They will spend most of their time reviewing the clinical records of the residents in the nursing home, checking meals that leave the kitchen to monitor the temperature of the meals, meeting with certain staff members when issues arise that require clarification, and meeting with residents and their family members to assess their views, feelings, etc. as it relates to the delivery of medical, social, dietary, activity, and spiritual services provided by the nursing home.

At the conclusion of the state survey, the surveyors will hold an "exit" meeting where they meet with management and non-management staff members of the nursing home to reveal the deficiencies they have discovered and the class of citations the nursing home can expect to be issued that range from minor to severe. If a citation is severe enough that a survey team has declared that the residents in a nursing home are in "eminent danger" and/or are receiving "sub-standard care" they can order the nursing home to close their doors and relocate their residents to other nursing homes in the local area. Should this happen to a nursing home, residents, family members, and staff are going to find their world turned upside down.

When a nursing home is issued citations, they are given a specific period of time to put their plan of correction in writing and deliver the plan of correction to the state survey team. They are also given a specific period of time in which to correct the issues that resulted in citations. A nursing home also has the right to a hearing to contest citations.

When citations in a nursing home are serious enough, the nursing home may lose their license that was in good standing and be issued a "conditional" license that will be in place until such a time as the state survey team feels that the noted citations have been corrected. When a nursing home is issued a conditional license, they may be subjected to more frequent surveys. For that fact, a state survey team is authorized to enter and inspect any nursing home at any given time.

Reality and human nature dictate that all employees in any area of expertise are not only capable of making mistakes, they will make mistakes. Given this, one can only expect a survey team to discover deficiencies as it relates to the delivery of services in nursing homes. When a state survey is completed, the results are required to be posted in a common area of a nursing home because residents, family members, visitors, and the general public have the right to inspect the results of the state survey. The bottom line is, nursing homes should be survey ready on any given day, not once a year.

Nursing homes are required to post the results of their most current survey in a common area of the facility where residents, family members, and visitors have the right to read the survey results. Prior to agreeing to be admitted to a nursing home, it would be wise to read the most current state survey as it relates to a nursing homes performance of delivery of health care services.

32

THERAPY

There are many senior citizens that are very active in sporting events. Over the years, knee, hip, and shoulder joints may become weaker and sustain injuries that will require surgery to repair. Without therapy, the healing process may take a very long time and the joints may not heal properly. While some patients may benefit from outpatient therapy, others require more intense therapy that is offered in long term care facilities.

There are three basic forms of therapy one can receive in a nursing home to include physical, occupational, and speech therapy. Physical therapists generally work with residents who experience musculoskeletal injuries and post orthopedic surgeries. They also treat injuries to tendons, ligaments, muscles, and bones. Residents in nursing homes that experience balance deficits would certainly benefit from a physical therapy regimen. They also work with resident's who have experienced a stroke resulting in balance problems, paralysis, and difficulty ambulating, that interfere with a resident's ability to function independently.

Occupational therapists work with residents as it relates to activities of daily living such as bathing, dressing, toileting, hygiene, and grooming. Residents that have had surgery and/or suffer some form of paralysis related to a stoke or heart attack will certainly have difficulty completing tasks that they once considered quite basic, and are now considered quite challenging. Occupational therapists also conduct evaluations of a resident's home environment to assess the safety of the environment and to suggest recommendations on how to alter an environment to make it safer for a resident to return home, as well as, promoting functional independence in a home environment.

Residents that now require a wheelchair for mobility will have to restructure their home environment to navigate around furniture and other articles in their home. They may now require grab bars in the tub or shower so a resident may be able to bathe independently.

Speech therapists are able to diagnose and treat speech and language disorders as well as assist residents with cognitive communication. Difficulty swallowing and/or communication may result from a stroke and/or diseases such as Parkinson's disease and Multiple Sclerosis. Some symptoms of a swallowing deficit may include having difficulty initiating swallowing after chewing food, may experience choking or coughing on foods, aspiration pneumonia related to liquids, and may experience weight loss and/or dehydration.

As a resident in a nursing home that is having difficulty swallowing, their physician may order a Modified Barium Swallow study to be performed on a resident. During this procedure, varying consistencies of food and liquids mixed with barium sulfate are given to a patient and the patient is x-rayed to hopefully determine the etiology and the severity of the swallowing disorder.

Speech therapists also advise staff in dining areas of nursing homes on what to look for in residents that may have swallowing deficits such as coughing or choking and educates staff related to correct posture during meals, the consistency of foods and liquids, and the size of mouthfuls a resident can safely swallow.

As a resident in a nursing home that is receiving any and/or all of the therapies outlined above, you may find therapy very time consuming, difficult to perform, and painful at times, however, before you decide to refuse therapy, inquire of the therapist as to the long term effects of your refusal of therapy.

33

VALUABLES

When a resident is admitted to a nursing home, a written inventory should be taken of all their possessions and the resident and/or their family should be given a copy of the written inventory. Remember, every time you bring new articles into a nursing home for a resident such as clothes, furniture and jewelry, be sure to meet with the unit secretary to ensure that the new articles are recorded on the resident's possession record and the staff member recording the new articles signs the form as the individual who recorded the items.

As a resident or family member and are having possessions inventoried, do not become upset if the unit secretary describes your jewelry as gold or silver in color with a certain colored stone. They are instructed by management to describe a resident's jewelry in such a fashion because a nursing home has no way of being assured that the jewelry is actually gold or silver, or in fact, contains precious, valuable gems unless presented with an appraisal of the jewelry. If a resident's jewelry being brought into a nursing home requires a written appraisal, it would be wise for an Administrator to suggest that the resident release the jewelry to a person of their choice. It is very important that you inquire, during the admissions process, as to whether the nursing home is financially responsible for missing valuables.

As a resident in a nursing home, do not bring very valuable items, jewelry, etc. to the nursing home with you. As a resident and you do not have family members in the local area who can store and protect your valuables, request that the nursing home place your valuables in their safe and be sure to obtain a receipt.

I often encouraged family members of residents that are cognitively impaired to replace their loved ones heirloom/valuable jewelry with costume jewelry that resembles the original that your loved one can continue to enjoy wearing and you do not have to worry about missing valuables. If a special occasion arises, you can always bring valuable jewelry to the nursing home for a resident to wear but remember to take it home with you when the evening has come to a close.

As a resident, do not keep sums of money on your person or in your room. Most nursing homes have what are referred to as "resident's accounts" where resident's can deposit money for safe keeping and withdraw money when the need arises.

34

VISITING

Visiting hours in nursing homes are generally quite liberal. Upon admission, do not be surprised if staff suggests that family and friends not visit the resident for at least one week after admission so that the resident may have adequate time to adjust to placement in the nursing home. Many residents admitted to nursing homes often feel abandoned by family members who have had to place them in a nursing home. It may be unrealistic at times for a nursing home to expect a resident to make an adequate adjustment to placement when their feelings of abandonment are exacerbated because the staff requested they not receive visitors for at least a week after admission.

I feel a compromise would better suit a resident and their family and friends if staff would suggest that they limit their visiting during the first week of admission. When visiting your loved one or a friend in a nursing home and they start verbally berating you and/or blaming you for them being in a nursing home, limiting your visiting may also be beneficial.

As family and friends of a resident in a nursing home you are going to have your own emotional issue to cope with so do not permit a resident to verbally abuse you and/or make you feel guilty for their placement in a nursing home.

AFTERWORD

My motivation for writing this book arose out of my frustration as a Social Worker in nursing homes as it relates to assisting newly admitted residents with making an adequate adjustment to long term placement. With caseloads of over one hundred residents, it was quite difficult to perform this responsibility adequately and nursing home management did not present as sympathetic to this issue. Therefore, I thought I would write a book to assist residents in nursing homes to make an adequate adjustment to placement and to ensure that their rights are protected.

Now that you have read my book you can now see many issues that may or will arise as a result of being admitted to a nursing home. You now know how to identify and address problems as they arise and to ensure that your rights are respected and protected by the staff in a nursing home and that you will receive the best care possible.

Given the amount of information covered in my book it may be difficult for some folks to retain all the information, therefore, it was my intention for my book to be a reference manual that is meant to be reviewed again and again as problems arise.

It is my hope that should you ever have to be admitted to a nursing home, you will face a minimum of problems.

978-0-595-45317-7
0-595-45317-1